Occupational Epidemiology

Author

Richard R. Monson, M.D., Sc.D.
Department of Epidemiology
Harvard University
School of Public Health
Boston, Massachusetts

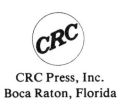

CRC Press, Inc.
Boca Raton, Florida

Library of Congress Cataloging in Publication Data

Monson, Richard R.
Occupational epidemiology.

  Bibliography: p.
  Includes index.
  1. Occupational diseases. 2. Epidemiology.
I. Title. [DNLM : 1. Epidemiology methods.
WA950M775o]
RC964.M66   616,9'803'072   79-27046
ISBN 0-8493-5793-4

   Direct all inquiries to CRC Press, Inc., 2000 Corporate Blvd., N.W., Boca Raton, Florida, 33431.

© 1980 by CRC Press, Inc.
Second Printing, 1981
Third Printing, 1982
Fourth Printing, 1983
Fifth Printing, 1984
Sixth Printing, 1985
Seventh Printing, 1986
Eighth Printing, 1987

International Standard Book Number 0-8493-5793-4

Library of Congress Card Number 79-27046
Printed in the United States

PREFACE

Epidemiology as a word dates back to Hippocrates. His writings describe the occurrence of acute epidemic diseases in various populations. Epidemiology as a discipline has no precise beginning. Physicians concerned with the ravages upon populations of influenza, cholera, plague, and other infectious diseases were the first epidemiologists. Because of this concern, epidemiology gradually evolved into the study of the occurrence of infectious disease in human populations.

As early as 1662, however, a different aspect of the study of human populations emerged. A London haberdasher, John Graunt, published in that year his *Natural and Political Observations Made upon the Bills of Mortality.* In this book Graunt observed that data from populations exhibit a numerical regularity from year to year. Because of this regularity, he reasoned that data collected for political or administrative reasons could be used to gain knowledge about human behavior and illnesses. This recognition forms the basis of the epidemiology of today.

There are two distinct types of departments of epidemiology in today's universities and at least two types of epidemiologist. Infectious disease comprises one major subject matter area in epidemiology; noninfectious or chronic disease comprises a second. In some locations these two types of epidemiologist work together closely while elsewhere there is little interaction. Because of these two faces of epidemiology, different cultures exist within the field. Each culture has its own way of thinking and its own terminology. This has led to disagreement over the words as well as the concepts of epidemiology.

My training and work has been in chronic disease epidemiology. My experience is in evaluating the associations between exposures that may last a number of years and diseases that have insidious onsets. The time between first exposure and first manifestation of disease may be many years. Evaluation of these associations forms the basis of occupational epidemiology.

The methods used in occupational epidemiology differ only in emphasis from those used in chronic disease epidemiology. Consequently, in the first section of this book a general review of epidemiologic methods is provided. As examples, in addition to studies of occupation and disease, data relating radiation or medications to disease are used. Each is a useful model for occupational exposures. Radiation in high doses is known to be harmful; in low doses controversy over its harmfulness exists. Medications or drugs, on the other hand, are widely used in human populations and are generally believed to be beneficial. However, it is becoming apparent that long-term usage of drugs can lead to serious chronic diseases. The analogy between such exposures and occupational exposures is apparent.

The subject matter of occupational health includes the subject matter of occupational epidemiology. However, occupational medicine has developed much in the manner of infectious disease epidemiology. Occupational health physicians over the years have dealt primarily with acute diseases resulting from short-term exposures to physical and chemical agents. Their emphasis has been on the prevention and cure of these illnesses. No elaborate scientific methodology had to be developed to assess whether exposure to dust led to acute bronchitis. The efforts of the occupational health physician could be directed toward treating the bronchitis and reducing the dust exposure. However, a practicing physician has little opportunity to assess whether 20 years of working with benzene leads to leukemia. The exposure may have produced no intolerable symptoms; the disease may not have developed until 10 years after the exposure has stopped.

I have written this book for the occupational health professional in the hope that the union of epidemiology and occupational health will be seen as a natural one. However, I believe there is a wider audience: students in occupational health, industrial hygiene, or epidemiology programs may benefit from a widening of their horizons; students in medical school may find an aspect of clinical medicine or research that is both stimulating and beneficial to society.

I thank Dr. Brian MacMahon and Dr. James Whittenberger for their support. I am indebted to Trudie Crowley, Doris Carmo, Lori Jackson, Mary O'Loughlin, and Virginia Ruggiero for their deciphering and typing ability and to Margrieta Zalkalns for her graphic skills.

THE AUTHOR

Richard R. Monson, M.D., Sc.D., is Professor of Epidemiology, Harvard School of Public Health, Boston, Massachusetts. Dr. Monson received his B.S. in chemistry from North Dakota State University in 1958, his M.D. from Harvard Medical School, and his Sc.M. and Sc.D. in epidemiology and biostatistics from Harvard School of Public Health.

Dr. Monson is a member of the Society for Epidemiologic Research. He is the author of over fifty papers in the fields of occupational and environmental epidemiology. His current research centers on the relationship between the workplace, the environment, and disease.

To Pat

TABLE OF CONTENTS

Chapter 1
A HISTORY OF EPIDEMIOLOGY

I. JOHN GRAUNT

As indicated in the preface, modern epidemiologic thinking dates to John Graunt. Around 1532, in London, a weekly tally was begun of the number of persons who died from various causes.[1] This was the era of the plague, and the town council apparently felt it to be of value to keep a count of the number of persons dying from the plague and from other causes.

On and off for over 100 years these Bills of Mortality were collected. For reasons not known, John Graunt's interest was aroused. He writes to a member of the Privie Council:[2]

Now having (I know not by what accident) engaged my thoughts upon the *Bills of Mortality*, and so far succeeded therein, as to have reduced several great confused *Volumes* into a few perspicuous *Tables*, and abridged such *Observations* as naturally flowed from them, into a few succinct *Paragraphs*, without any long series of *multiloquious Deductions*, I have presumed to sacrifice these my small, but first publish'd, *Labours* into your Lordship, as unto whose benigne acceptance of some other of my *Papers*, even the Birth of these is due; . . . I hoped it might not be ungratefull to your Lordship, to see unto how much profit that one Talent might be improved, beside the many curiosities concerning the waxing and waning of Diseases.

In this introductory paragraph, Graunt recognizes several of the elementary principles of epidemiology:

1. Voluminous data should be reduced to a few perspicuous tables.
2. The description of these data should be brief.
3. The interpretation of these data should be conservative.
4. Profit may be gained by observing data arising from populations.

The Bills were collected as follows:

When any one dies, then, either by tolling, or ringing of a Bell, or by bespeaking of a Grave of the *Sexton,* the same is known to the *Searchers,* corresponding with the said *Sexton.* The *Searchers* hereupon (who are antient matrons, sworn to their office) repair to the place, where the dead Corps lies, and by view of the same, and by other enquiries, they examine by what *Disease,* or *Casualty* the Corps died.[2]

This procedure has aspects similar to that used in completing the death certificate. An opinion of a physician is recorded as to the cause of death. In general, information from the autopsy is not entered onto the death certificate. Yet, Graunt recognized as does today's epidemiologist that, in spite of the lack of precision as to the definition of the disease that led to death, information is nonetheless obtainable from deceased persons.

Graunt was the first to recognize that there were more male than female births:

There have been Buried from the year 1628, to the year 1662, *exclusive,* 209 436 *Males,* and but 190 474 *Females:* but it will be objected, that in *London* it may indeed be so, though otherwise elsewhere; because *London* is the great Stage and Shop of business, wherein the *Masculine Sex* bears the greatest part. But we Answer, That there have been also *Christened* within the same time, 139 782 *Males,* and but 130 866 Females, . . ., What the Causes hereof are, we shall not trouble ourselves to conjecture, as in other Cases, onely we shall desire, that Travellers would enquire whether it be the same in other Countries.[2]

In this passage Graunt observes more male deaths than female deaths, questions the validity as to interpretation, and reinforces the belief that there are more males than females by counting the number of births. However, he displays proper conservatism by recommending that this phenomenon in London be searched for elsewhere.

Graunt makes observations on morbidity as well as mortality:

> It appearing, that there were fourteen men to thirteen women, and that they die in the same proportion also, yet I have heard *Physicians* say, that they have two woman Patients to one man, . . . Now, from this it should follow, that more women should die than men . . . but this must be salved, either by alledging, that the *Physicians* cure those Sicknesses, so as few more die, then if none were sick; or else that men, being more intemperate than women, die as much by reason of their Vices, as the women do by the Infirmities of their *Sex*.[2]

Here, Graunt tries to reconcile common knowledge with data. If both the physicians and his data are correct, several explanations are possible. Graunt does not conclude that either explanation is possible; he merely offers alternates. Such behavior reflects the caution that is needed in the interpretation of epidemiologic data. The numbers may or may not reflect facts. More than one explanation usually is possible. The role of the epidemiologist is to collect the data in as accurate a manner as possible and to suggest possible explanations. More definite interpretation must be provided by persons who can judge not only the data but also the data collector.

Graunt provided the foundation for the development of the life table. Here, he overstepped his basic observational method and constructed a theoretical model:[2]

> Whereas we have found, that of 100 quick Conceptions about 36 of them die before they be six years old, and that perhaps but one surviveth 76, we, having seven *Decads* between six and 76, we sought six mean proportional numbers between 64, the remainder, living at six years, and the one, which survives 76, and finde, that the numbers following are practically near enough to the truth;

Viz. of 100 there dies	The fourth 6
within the first six years 36	The next 4
the next ten years, or	The next 3
Decad 24	The next 2
The second *Decad* 15	The next 1
The third *Decad* 09	

Graunt may be forgiven this excursion into theory, for he states that the facts lie near enough to the truth. There has always existed in humans a desire to discover the natural laws and formulas that govern human existence. As a group, epidemiologists also seek these laws. However, much of the data available to Graunt as well as to today's epidemiologist is flawed. To base natural laws on such data is frequently an over-extension of the possible.

Finally, Graunt asks "to what purpose tends all this laborious buzzling, and groping?" He answers: "I conclude, That a clear knowledge of all these particulars, and many more, whereat I have shot but at rovers, is necessary in order to good, certain, and easie Government . . . But whether the knowledge thereof be necessary to many, or fit for others . . . I leave to consideration."[2]

A contemporary of Graunt, Sir William Petty, termed the science of Graunt "Political Arithmetic".[3] This term is a good description of today's epidemiology. Much of the data manipulation that epidemiologists do requires a fourth grade education in arithmetic. However, the wisdom as to the validity of the data and the conservatism of interpretation requires persons with a keen political sense.

II. WILLIAM FARR

For 200 years after Graunt, there was no expansion upon his ideas. Medical historians attribute this to Syndenham, a contemporary of Graunt. Syndenham was a prominent physician and is recognized as being the first to maintain sequential medical records on his patients. However, he taught that disease was not only related to the symptoms in the patient but to the seasons and the "epidemic constitutions". His teaching derived from the metaphysics of Hippocrates rather than from the arithmetic of Graunt.

Syndenham, one of the most accurate of medical writers, in speaking of small-pox, employed such terms as these: (1661) "It prevailed a little, but disappeared again." — (1667—9) "The small-pox was more prevalent in town for the first two years of this constitution than I ever remember it to have been" . . . these terms admit of no strict comparison with each other; for it is difficult to say in which year the small-pox was most fatal, and impossible to compare Syndenham's experience thus expressed with the experience of other writers in other places and other ages; for "prevailed a little", "raged with violence", and similar terms, may imply either that small-pox destroyed 1, or 2, or 5, or 10 per cent of the population. The superior precision of numerical expressions is illustrated by a comparison of Syndenham's phrases with the London bills of mortality in the same years, as seen in Table 1.1.

The 1,987 deaths from small-pox in 1668, and the 951 deaths from that disease in the year following, express the relative intensity of small-pox in distinct terms. The method of the parish clerks, although imperfectly carried out, was the best.[4]

These observations were written by William Farr, the Superintendent of the Statistical Department of the General Register Office in 19th century Great Britain. Farr was a physician with an interest in numbers — the perfect description of an early epidemiologist. In 1837, the annual registration of the numbers and causes of deaths in England was begun, and in 1839 Farr was appointed Compiler of Abstracts. For over 30 years he was responsible for the yearly tally of causes of deaths.

The organization of a continuing system of recording information on mortality was Farr's contribution to epidemiology. Graunt recognized the value of data that had been assembled on human populations. Farr took the next step and set up a system for the routine compilation of such data.

William Farr, however, was more than a dull compiler of dull data. He recognized that the data derived from human lives and that the data could be used to learn about human existence:

The primary object is to determine what the death-toll is at the several ages, and what the causes of the loss of life are, under different circumstances. The importance of this determination will become apparent by enumerating some of the relations the mortality bears to other orders of facts. There is a relation betwixt death and sickness; and to every death from every cause there is an average number of attacks of sickness, and a specific number of persons incapacitated for work. Death is the extinction of pain. There is a relation betwixt death, health, and energy of body and mind. There is a relation betwixt death, birth, and marriage. There is a relation betwixt death and national primacy: numbers turn the tide in the struggle of populations, and the most mortal die out.

If the latent cause of epidemics cannot be discovered, the mode in which it operates may be investigated. The laws of its action may be determined by observation, as well as the circumstances in which epidemics arise, or by which they can be controlled.

The deaths and causes of death are scientific facts which admit of numerical analysis; and science has nothing to offer more inviting in speculation than the laws of vitality, the variations of those laws in the two sexes at different ages, and the influence of civilization, occupation, locality, seasons, and other physical agencies, either in generating diseases and inducing death, or in improving the public health.[4]

Farr recognized, as did Graunt, that there was a regularity in the data arising from the observation of human populations. He further recognized that an ultimate understanding of the reasons for the numbers may not be possible. However, only by col-

Table 1.1
DEATHS FROM SMALLPOX IN
LONDON

Year	Deaths
1666	38
1667	1196
1668	1987
1669	951
1670	1465
1671	1465
1672	696
1673	1116
1674	853

lecting the numbers and evaluating them can one gain understanding of the forces that cause disease.

The first systematic evaluation of the relationship between occupation and cause of death was instituted by Farr. He recognized that on a death certificate neither the occupation nor the cause of death were precise statements of the person's life work or his reason for dying. Nonetheless, he did not discard the information because of this imprecision. An early 20th century epidemiologist, Major Greenwood, writes:

This willingness to accept what he could get was perhaps the most important of Farr's virtues. Wishing to study the influence of occupational environment upon health, he adopted the simple plan of relating the deaths in the census year to the population as enumerated in occupational groups. Any critically minded man could point out objections to this method. The occupation recorded in a death certificate is the occupation known to the dead man's relations who from ignorance or snobbishness may report a designation altogether different from that which the living man would return in the census form. Then there is the difficulty — which still confronts us — of distinguishing between the industrial and the occupational point of view in *both* sets of data . . . His survey . . . was less elaborate than those now attempted . . . but it is always directly to the point: "Tool, file, and sawmakers have among them the grinders who suffer so much from sharp particles of stone and steel inhaled into the lungs; their mortality is still high, and at the ages 45 to 65 excessive . . . The earthenware manufacture is one of the unhealthiest trades in the country. At the age of joining it is low; but the mortality after the age of 35 approaches double the average; it is excessively high; it exceeds the mortality of publicans. What can be done to save the men dying so fast in the potteries and engaged in one of our most useful manufactures?"[5]

As can be seen, Farr's work laid the ground for today's mortality studies of employed groups. The fact that workers in the earthenware industry had a mortality double the average is to say that their SMR (standardized mortality ratio) was 200. William Farr is to be thanked for this contribution to occupational epidemiology.

It must not be thought that Farr was a person who simply did the best he could with imperfect data. He also had a critical side and would point out error where it existed. Again in the occupational setting, an easy comparison was the mean age at death of persons employed in different industries. Farr pointed out the potential fallacy of such computations:

As the mean duration of life, technically called the expectation of life, differs very widely from the "mean age at death", and from some estimates which have been made of the relative health of different portions of the population, it may be right, before I close this Report, to point out the errors into which inquiries are liable to fall in reasoning upon the age at death; or, which is the same thing, constructing life tables from the deaths alone . . . It has been somewhere stated that the "mean age at death" of dress makers is exceeding low, and this has been adduced as a proof of the destructive effects of their employment. If the inquiries had been extended to boarding schools, or to the boys at Christ's Hospital, the "mean age at death'' would have been found still lower. Mr. Grainger states, in his interesting Report, that the majority of dress-makers are between the ages of 16 and 26; and it is understood that if they die after they marry they are not often designated by that title in the register. This source of error and the increase of population will be found to affect the estimate of the influence of other occupations. That the lives of dress-makers are very much shortened by the severe hardships and ignorant mistreatment to which they are exposed cannot be doubted; but false arguments injure instead of aiding their cause.[4]

The potential fallacy of computing the mean age of death of different groups and using it to estimate the shortening effects of occupation upon life was recognized by Farr over 100 years ago. Yet reports still occur in which this technique is used.[6,7]

As noted, Farr's principal contribution was the setting up of a system for the routine collection and maintenance of data on the population of Great Britain. This enabled future epidemiologists to use the data on past populations. In Farr's case, the data he collected were used by a contemporary, John Snow, to study the reasons for the epidemics of cholera in England.

Farr noted that there was an association between cholera mortality and elevation above sea level. Persons living at higher elevations died less frequently from cholera than did persons living at the level of the Thames. He published the data presented in Table 1.2.

Farr noted that the districts differed not only in their elevation, but also in their water supply and in the wealth of the inhabitants. Thus he recognized that the association between elevation and cholera mortality need not necessarily be regarded as a causal association. However, as did Graunt, Farr ventured a bit too far into theory in his ''Calculated Series''. The desire to explain data on the basis of some underlying natural law could not be resisted by even the most pragmatic of pioneers in epidemiology.

III. JOHN SNOW

John Snow is perhaps the best known person who is regarded as a founder of today's epidemiology. His work was recognized as being important in London in 1855 and is a mandatory reference in most epidemiology texts of today. This recognition is deserved; however, without the insights of John Graunt and William Farr, John Snow may not have been able to take the next step.

As noted, William Farr had published data showing that cholera mortality was inversely related to the elevation at which people lived. Starting with this observation, John Snow collected further data which showed that the explanation could be found in the water supply of the various districts. Thus he was able to demonstrate an immediate utility to epidemiologic data and to make recommendations that led to the prevention of cholera. It is perhaps in the utility of Snow's work that his fame lies rather than in the methods he used. His methods, however, deserve consideration.

Snow was a practicing physician. Through his contact with cholera patients, he made a number of observations:

It never attacks the crews of ships going from a country free from cholera, to one where the disease is prevailing, till they have entered a port, or had intercourse with the shore.

Besides the facts above mentioned, which prove that cholera is transmitted from person to person, there are others which show, first, that being present in the same room with a patient, and attending on him, do not necessarily expose a person to the morbid poison; and, secondly, that it is not always requisite that a person should be very near a cholera patient in order to take the disease, as the morbid matter producing it may be transmitted to a distance.

A consideration of the pathology of cholera is capable of indicating to us the manner in which the disease is communicated . . . I conclude that cholera invariably commences with the affection of the alimentary

Table 1.2
CHOLERA DEATH RATE IN 19TH CENTURY LONDON ACCORDING TO ELEVATION OF RESIDENCE ABOVE SEA LEVEL

Elevation of districts in feet	Number of terrace from bottom	Deaths from cholera in 10,000 inhabitants	Calculated series		
Under 20	1	102	102/1	=	102
20—40	2	65	102/2	=	51
40—60	3	34	102/3	=	34
60—80	4	27	102/4	=	26
80—100	5	22	102/5	=	20
100—120	6	17	102/6	=	17
340—360	18	7	102/18	=	6

canal . . . there can be no doubt that these symptoms depend upon the exudation from the mucous membrane, which is soon afterwards copiously evacuated . . . there is often a way open for (cholera) to extend itself more widely, and to reach the well-to-do classes of the community; I allude to the mixture of the cholera evacuations with the water used for drinking and culinary purposes, either by permeating the ground, and getting into wells, or by running along channels and sewers into the rivers from which entire towns are sometimes supplied with water.

The most terrible outbreak of cholera which ever occurred in this kingdom, is probably that which took place in Broad Street, Golden Square, and the adjoining streets, a few weeks ago . . . As soon as I became acquainted with the situation and extent of the irruption of cholera, I suspected some contamination of the water of the much-frequented street-pump in Broad Street . . . On proceeding to the spot, I found that nearly all the deaths had taken place within a short distance of the pump . . . I had an interview with the Board of Guardians of St. James's parish, on the evening of Thursday, 7th September, and represented the above circumstances to them. In consequence of what I said, the handle of the pump was removed on the following day.[8]

This account of Snow's experience with cholera could no doubt have been written by other physicians of the day. Snow basically writes of impressions gained through his years of clinical experience. He makes a recommendation based on his deductions and observes that cholera diminishes. There is little use of data accumulated on human populations in his relating of his experiences.

John Snow's contribution to the history of epidemiology lies in the next steps he took. He was not satisfied that the epidemic at Broad Street had subsided. Rather, he wished to show beyond doubt that cholera in London was associated with the source of drinking water. From data supplied by William Farr, Snow constructed Table 1.3 (modified).

Snow observed that the death rate from cholera was lowest in districts partially supplied by the Lambeth Company. This company obtained its water from the Thames above London, where it was "quite free from the sewage of London".

Snow's next step was to tally cholera deaths in subdistricts where the water supply could be more precisely specified. He focussed on the difference in mortality rates between the subdistricts supplied by the Lambeth Company and those supplied by the Southwark and Vauxhall (Table 1.4).

It seems clear that living in subdistricts supplied by the Southwark and Vauxhall water supply had something to do with dying from cholera. This, however, was not strong enough evidence for Snow. There were differences between these two areas other than water supply that might account for the difference in the cholera rates. Fortunately, there was one region in London that was supplied jointly by the two companies.

Table 1.3
CHOLERA DEATH RATE IN LONDON
ACCORDING TO WATER COMPANY
SUPPLYING DISTRICT OF RESIDENCE

Water company	Population	Deaths by cholera	Deaths in 100,000 inhabitants
(1) Southwark and Vauxhall (2) Kent	17,805	19	107
Southwark and Vauxhall	118,267	111	94
(1) Lambeth and (2) Southwark and Vauxhall	346,363	211	61

Table 1.4
CHOLERA DEATH RATE IN LONDON
ACCORDING TO WATER COMPANY
SUPPLYING SUBDISTRICT OF RESIDENCE

Water company	Population in 1851	Deaths from cholera	Deaths in 100,000 living
Southwark and Vauxhall	167,654	192	114
Both companies	301,149	182	60
Lambeth	14,632	0	0

Although the facts shown in the above table afford very strong evidence of the powerful influence which the drinking of water containing the sewage of a town exerts over the spread of cholera, when that disease is present, yet the question does not end here; for the intermixing of the water supply of the Southwark and Vauxhall Company with that of the Lambeth Company, over an extensive part of London, admitted of the subject being sifted in such a way as to yield the most incontrovertible proof on one side or the other. In the subdistricts enumerated in the above table as being supplied by both Companies, the mixing of the supply is of the most intimate kind. The pipes of each Company go down all the streets, and into nearly all the courts and alleys. A few houses are supplied by one Company and a few by the other, according to the decision of the owner or occupier at that time when the Water Companies were in active competition. In many cases a single house has a supply different from that on either side. Each company supplies both rich and poor, both large houses and small; there is no difference either in the condition or occupation of the persons receiving the water of the different Companies. Now it must be evident that, if the diminution of cholera, in the districts partly supplied with the improved water, depended on this supply, the houses receiving it would be the houses enjoying the whole benefit of the diminution of the malady, whilst the houses supplied with the water from Battersea Fields would suffer the same mortality as they would if the improved supply did not exist at all. As there is no difference whatever, either in the houses or the people receiving the supply of the two Water Companies, or in any of the physical conditions with which they are surrounded, it is obvious that no experiment could have been devised which would more thoroughly test the effect of water supply on the progress of cholera than this, which circumstances placed ready made before the observer.

The experiment, too, was on the grandest scale. No fewer than three hundred thousand people of both sexes, of every age and occupation, and of every rank and station, from gentlefolks down to the very poor, were divided into two groups without their choice, and, in most cases, without their knowledge; one group being supplied with water containing the sewage of London, and, amongst it, whatever might have come from the cholera patients, the other group having water quite free from such impurity.

Table 1.5
CHOLERA DEATH RATE IN LONDON
ACCORDING TO WATER COMPANY
SUPPLYING HOUSE OF RESIDENCE

Water company	Number of houses	Deaths from cholera	Deaths in each 10,000 houses
Southwark and Vauxhall	40,046	1263	315
Lambeth	26,107	98	37
Rest of London	256,423	1422	59

To turn this grand experiment to account, all that was required was to learn the supply of water to each individual house where a fatal attack of cholera might occur . . .

I was desirous of making the investigation myself, in order that I might have the most satisfactory proof of the truth or fallacy of the doctrine which I had been advocating for five years. I had no reason to doubt the correctness of the conclusions I had drawn from the great number of facts already in my possession, but I felt the circumstance of the cholera-poison passing down the sewers of a great river, and being distributed through miles of pipes, and yet producing its specific effects, was a fact of so startling a nature, and of so vast importance to the community, that it could not be too rigidly examined, or established on too firm a basis.[8]

By walking from house to house, Snow obtained the name of the water company supplying each house where a fatal case of cholera occurred. From routine data supplied by the water companies, he counted the total number of houses in each district supplied by each company. Based on these data, Snow drew up Table 1.5.

Thus Snow was able to provide further evidence that water supplied by the Southwark and Vauxhall Company was associated with death from cholera. This account has been called a "natural experiment" because there was essentially random allocation of water (and of cholera bacteria) to a portion of persons living in a defined area of London. Snow recognized the value of such a situation and took the necessary steps to collect the needed information.

This study of John Snow is a model of the observations that the epidemiologists of today try to make:

1. He recognized an association between exposure and disease (water company and cholera mortality).
2. He formed a hypothesis: sewage in the water causes cholera.
3. He collected substantiating information for his hypothesis: in subdistricts supplied by only one company, the association was stronger.
4. He recognized an alternate explanation for the association: social class was associated both with district of residence and with cholera.
5. He found a way to minimize the effects of this alternate explanation by comparing cholera rates according to water supply within rather than between neighborhoods.
6. He effectively minimized the collection of false information in that most persons were not aware of the name of their water company.

Most important, however, was the fact that Snow's work led to the prevention of cholera. Whether this possibility was a motivating factor to Snow is uncertain. Perhaps it was obvious to him at the time that if he could convince others of the correctness of his hypothesis, mortality from cholera could be reduced. While this is the ultimate goal of most medical research, the immediacy of success is not always apparent to the epidemiologist of today. Consider, for example, cigarette smoking and lung cancer.

IV. CIGARETTES

Between the middle of the 19th century and the middle of the 20th century, epidemiology progressed slowly. Much attention was directed toward the semitheoretical study of how "epidemics" occurred in animal populations. Based on observations made on the spread of an infectious illness in a captive animal population, models were constructed and predictions were made on how illness spread in humans. This work was primarily relevant to infectious disease epidemiology; few of the methods or models have applicability in today's chronic disease or occupational epidemiology.

As World War II was ending, it was becoming apparent to physicians that more and more men were being seen with lung cancer. Before 1940, cancer of the lung was a medical curiosity. The examination of the reason for this increase in lung cancer provides a useful focus on the beginning of chronic disease epidemiology as it is practiced today.

Around 1950, a number of studies were begun to study the reason for this increase in the rate of lung cancer. Not surprisingly, cigarette smoking was a prime suspect. Two types of studies were therefore designed: in one, persons with and without lung cancer were asked about past habits, including smoking; in the second type of study, smokers and nonsmokers were followed for a period of time and the rates of development of a variety of diseases, including lung cancer, were measured. These two study types, case-control and cohort, are illustrative of the studies being conducted by today's epidemiologists. In a case-control study, factors associated with one or more diseases are determined. In a cohort study, diseases associated with one or more factors are determined.

A. Doll and Hill: Case-Control Study[9]

In 1947, an investigation was planned "to determine whether patients with carcinoma of the lung differed materially from other persons in respect to their smoking habits." Patients enrolled in the study included those admitted to a hospital in London with carcinoma of the lung, stomach, colon, or rectum. Also, a number of patients without cancer were included. Interviews were conducted with these patients and questions were asked about their past smoking habits.

If one considers only the patient with lung cancer and those without cancer, the results can be presented as in Table 1.6. It can be seen that 97% of persons with lung cancer were cigarette smokers and only 92% of persons with other diseases were smokers. Conversely, it may be stated that 3% of persons with lung cancer were nonsmokers in contrast to 8% of persons with other diseases.

These data must be interpreted. The numbers by themselves give no hint as to the reason for the difference in percentages. Questions that might be asked include:

1. Were the criteria for entrance into the study the same for the two groups of patients?
2. Do the persons with lung cancer and those without lung cancer differ in any way other than in their disease and their smoking habits?
3. Was the information on smoking habits collected in a similar way for cases and controls?
4. Did the authors have any personal interest as to the results of the study?
5. Is the difference in percentage of smokers large enough to be meaningful?

Table 1.6
RELATIONSHIP BETWEEN CIGARETTE SMOKING AND LUNG CANCER IN DOLL AND HILL'S CASE-CONTROL STUDY

	Lung cancer	
Cigarette smoker	Yes	No
Yes	688	650
No	21	59
Total	709	709
Percentage smoker	97	92

These and other questions must be asked about all epidemiologic studies. These questions are similar to those raised by John Graunt, William Farr, and John Snow. It is not enough to collect data on exposure and disease in a human population. Thought must be given as to possible alternate explanations of any association between exposure and disease that is found.

Doll and Hill asked questions and provided alternate explanations:

1. Could (the association) be due to an unrepresentative sample of patients with carcinoma of the lung or to a choice of a control series which was not truly comparable?
2. Could (the association) have been produced by an exaggeration of their smoking habits by patients who thought they had an illness which could be attributed to smoking?
3. Could (the association) be produced by a bias on the part of the interviewers in taking and interpreting the histories?
4. The association would occur if carcinoma of the lung caused people to smoke or if both attributes were end-results of a common cause.

After due consideration of alternate explanations, Doll and Hill "conclude that smoking is a factor, and an important factor, in the production of carcinoma of the lung . . . As to the nature of the carcinogen we have no evidence."

B. Doll and Hill — Cohort Study[10,11]

In 1951 a questionnaire was sent to all British physicians inquiring about their smoking habits. Over the next 25 years death certificates were collected whenever a physician died. The number of diseases recorded on the death certificates were related to the smoking habits of the physician.

This study is an example of the second type of epidemiologic study in common use today — the cohort study. Where in a case-control study the investigator starts with persons with and without some disease, in a cohort study the investigator starts with persons with and without some exposure. Case-control studies take a relatively short time to complete, since past history of exposure is the only information that is collected. Many cohort studies take a relatively long time to complete, since the occur-

Table 1.7
RELATIONSHIP BETWEEN CIGARETTE
SMOKING AND LUNG CANCER IN DOLL
AND HILL'S COHORT STUDY

Cigarette habit	Cases of lung cancer/100,000/year
Current smoker	104
Former smoker	43
Nonsmoker	10

rence of disease at some time in the future must be recorded. This cohort study, which started in 1951, is still going on today.

If one considers only the data on cigarette smoking and lung cancer, the results can be presented as in Table 1.7. Again, an association is seen between the cigarette smoking and lung cancer. The death rate from lung cancer in smokers is ten times the rate in nonsmokers.

Interpretation of these data must follow a procedure similar to that used in interpreting data resulting from a case-control study. The same questions must be asked and the possibility of explanations other than cause must be considered.

These papers by Doll and Hill provide an important link between the early epidemiologists and those of today. The value of collecting data on human populations is linked to the methodologies of the case-control and cohort studies. The possibility of alternate explanations of any association was emphasized by Graunt, Farr, and Snow and needs to be reemphasized today. The general utility of nonexperimental methods has been and continues to be the basis for epidemiologic research.

V. THE COMPUTER

The two studies of Doll and Hill were started before the everyday use of the electronic computer. Some mechanized help was available, inasmuch as punch cards and card sorting machines had been in use since the late 19th century. However, in 1950 considerable hand work was necessary in the conduct of epidemiologic studies.

Epidemiology is the study of disease occurrence in human populations.[12] The pioneering work of Graunt was an analysis of 100 years of data collected for other reasons. The pioneering work of Farr was the development of a system for the routine collection of data on humans that eventually could be used by epidemiologists. The work of these two men focussed on the gradual accumulation of large amounts of data to be used for general epidemiologic purposes.

John Snow, however, needed specific data on individuals with cholera; he needed to know who supplied their water. The only way he could get this information was to go house-to-house and ask. No doubt he kept tablets of paper with home address and water supply listed on each line.

In analyzing the data collected, Snow and Doll and Hill in their first study had to do their computations using relatively simple methods. By 1976 in the second Doll and Hill study, however, 25 years of data had accumulated. Considerable data had been collected on smoking habits over the years for over 34,000 physicians. Analysis by hand clearly would have been difficult.

The explosion of epidemiologic studies since 1950 is directly related to the development of the computer. The ability to collect large amounts of data, to store these data on a computer tape, and to conduct extensive analyses of these data is the hallmark of epidemiology today. Whereas strong associations between exposure and disease can be detected using simple analyses of small amounts of data, weak associations require extensive analyses of data from a large number of persons. Further, as interest has developed in the development of diseases such as cancer twenty or more years after exposure to some chemical, the use of the computer has become indispensable for storage and analysis of data.

The use of the computer in epidemiology is not without potential problems. Yesterday's epidemiologist usually was directly involved in the design of studies and the collection of data. Because of this he was acutely aware of the deficiencies of the nonexperimental study of human populations and of the need for cautious interpretation of data. The epidemiologist of today may have access to data collected by others that are stored on a computer and ready for instant analysis. Any weakness inherent in the collection of the data may not be apparent. However, the need for the careful analysis and cautious interpretation of epidemiologic data is as necessary now as it was in 1662.

VI. OCCUPATION AND EPIDEMIOLOGY

The recent history of epidemiology has focussed around the hospital. It is here that persons with disease are to be found; it is logical that the search for the causes of disease be centered around hospitals.

Increasingly, however, epidemiologists are seeking to study exposed persons rather than diseased persons. The long term effects of exposure to some substance are clearly as important as the antecedents of some disease. Persons working in industry have daily contact with large numbers of exposures — chemicals, noise, dust, heat, trauma, physical exertion, radiation. Some of these exposures are known to cause disease in humans; others are known to be harmful to animals if given in high doses; still others have no known adverse effect.

It is logical that epidemiologists evaluate the effects on health of workers in industry. However, how should these evaluations proceed? Conducting case-control studies in hospital populations is logical because that is where persons with diseases congregate. Conducting cohort studies in industrial populations also is logical because that is where persons with exposures congregate. However, as illustrated by the cohort study of British physicians, 25 years or more may be needed to assess the long-term effects of some exposure.

For this reason, epidemiologists in occupational settings have a great concern with records. If one can find records on industrial populations dating back 30 to 50 years, one can define cohorts based in the past rather than in the present. Follow-up need not take 25 years. Also, today's occupational epidemiologists must be concerned about the future. The records and data of today must be maintained for the epidemiologists of tomorrow. In this way, any adverse effects of working in industry can be more readily detected and prevented.

REFERENCES

1. **Pearl, R.,** *Introduction to Medical Biometry and Statistics,* W. B. Saunders, Philadelphia, 1940, 27.
2. **Graunt, J.,** *Natural and Political Observations Made upon the Bills of Mortality,* Willcox, W. F., Ed., Johns Hopkins University Press, Baltimore, 1939.
3. **Dick, O. L.,** *Aubrey's Brief Lives,* University of Michigan Press, Ann Arbor, 1957, 114.
4. **Farr, W.,** *Vital Statistics: A Memorial Volume of Selections from the Reports and Writings of William Farr,* Humphreys, N. A., Ed., Office of the Sanitary Institute, London, 1885.

5. **Greenwood, M.** *The Medical Dictator and other Biographical Studies,* Williams and Norgate, London, 1936, 111.
6. **Luria, S. M.,** Average age at death of scientists in various specialities, *Public Health Rep.,* 84, 661, 1969.
7. Longevity of United States Senators, *Stat. Bull. Metrop. Life Insur. Co.,* 50, 2, 1969.
8. **Snow, J.,** *Snow on Cholera,* Hafner Publishing, New York, 1965.
9. **Doll, R. and Hill, A. B.,** Smoking and carcinoma of the lung, *Br. Med. J.,* 2, 739, 1950.
10. **Doll, R. and Hill, A. B.,** Mortality of doctors in relation to their smoking habits. A preliminary report, *Br. Med. J.,* 1, 1451, 1954.
11. **Doll, R. and Peto, R.,** Mortality in relation to smoking: 20 years' observations on male British doctors, *Br. Med. J.,* 2, 1525, 1976.
12. **MacMahon, B. and Pugh, T. F.,** *Epidemiology — Principles and Methods,* Little, Brown, Boston, 1970, 1.

General Epidemiology
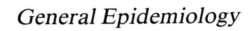

Chapter 2
THE NATURE OF EPIDEMIOLOGIC DATA

I. INTRODUCTION

Data on populations may come from a number of settings: examples of data include the number of male cats living in Boston in 1980, the annual rate of cancer in laboratory animals, the number of patrons at Fenway Park during the Yankee series, the percentage of white students in South Boston High School, the number of new epidemiologists who graduate each year, the percentage of livers at autopsy that show cirrhosis, the number of new cases of lung cancer among cigarette smokers each year, the rate of leukemia in rubber workers who have heavy solvent exposure compared to the rate of leukemia in workers who have no solvent exposure. Each of these measures has the common feature that a number is used. Numbers by themselves carry no information as to the source of the information. Therefore, there is more to epidemiology than the simple manipulation of data.

Data may be thought of as continuous or discrete. Examples of continuous data include height and weight, the price of meat, temperature, the capacity of a lung, the mortality rate in a population. Examples of discrete data include sex (male, female), religion, ethnic group, and the presence or absence of a specific disease. Epidemiologists use data that are discrete as well as data that are continuous.

The most basic setting giving rise to epidemiologic data is the evaluation of the occurrence of a disease in the presence of an exposure. The exposure may be present or absent and the disease may be present or absent. By cross-tabulating exposure vs. disease, any population may be divided into four parts: exposed and diseased, exposed and not diseased, not exposed and diseased, or not exposed and not diseased. In tabular form, this is called a fourfold table (Table 2.1).

Either discrete or continuous data can be put in the form of a fourfold table. For example, continuous data such as height and weight can be degraded into tall-short and heavy-light. Data on ethnicity and religion can be combined into Caucasian-other and Protestant-other. Information may be lost in creating a simple fourfold table from more complex data, but the information that remains is still valid.

While the fourfold table forms the basis for much of epidemiologic practice, its use is not limited to epidemiology. Most data can be made to conform to the fourfold table. Thus data from experiments on animals have the same appearance as data from observations on humans. Such data can be manipulated and analyzed irrespective of their source. However, in the interpretation of such analyses, consideration must be given to the source of the data.

II. SOURCES OF DATA

A. Animal Populations

In the search for causal agents, preventive agents, and curative agents, extensive experimental research is being done on animal populations. Data are gathered on the relation between exposure and disease or treatment and cure of disease. Such data can be put in the form of a fourfold table for analysis.

The characteristics of research on laboratory animals are such that the analysis and interpretation of data are relatively straightforward. These characteristics include:

Table 2.1
THE FOURFOLD TABLE

Disease

Exposure	Yes	No	Total
Yes	a	b	a + b
No	c	d	c + d
Total	a + c	b + d	a + b + c + d

1.   Laboratory animals tend to be inbred strains; therefore, there is relatively little variation in the genetic makeup among animals.
2.   Exposure or nonexposure to an agent is solely determined by the investigator; therefore, animals can be assigned at random to exposed or nonexposed groups.
3.   The entire life-span of the animal is under continuous observation; therefore, relatively precise measures of exposure and disease are possible.

In assessing the relationship or association between exposure and disease in animal populations, an investigator need consider only whether the rate of disease in the exposed group differs from the rate of disease in the nonexposed group for one of two reasons: chance or cause. Because of the inherent variability in biologic systems, no two experiments give the same results. The rate of cancer in one group of mice treated with a suspected carcinogen will usually differ from the rate in a second group of mice treated in a similar manner simply because of "chance". Therefore, if two groups of mice are treated with two different agents, the two rates may also differ because of chance.

The methods of statistics have been developed in such settings. All systems have a basic variability that makes replications of experiments differ from each other. There is a regularity in this variability, be it in a biologic system, a physical system, or a chemical system. Because of this regularity, one can predict with fair accuracy the degree of variability when a given experiment is repeated many times. In flipping a set of ten coins 100 times, one can predict that the most frequent result usually will be five heads and five tails. Next most frequent will be four heads and six tails or six heads and four tails. Only rarely will there be ten heads or ten tails. Formulas have been developed that predict with great accuracy the results of such trials. Theory and practice thus complement each other.

In animal systems, there is usually more variability in the results of repeated experiments. Even inbred mice have considerably more inherent variation from one mouse to another than do sets of pennies. However, in spite of this greater variability, the laws of probability are as applicable in experimental biologic settings as in experimental physical settings. This is because of the ability of the investigator to assign exposure randomly.

Tests of statistical significance have a general utility in such systems. In essence, these tests provide an estimate of the likelihood or probability that the results of a given experiment could have arisen by chance alone. Since the main alternative to a chance association between exposure and disease is a causal association, causal inferences may be made with reasonable assurance. Even in such relatively simple experimental situations, however, chance can never be ruled out absolutely as an explanation for an association.

Data resulting from nonexperimental studies on human populations frequently have the same appearance as data arising from experimental studies on animal populations. Therefore, investigators frequently analyze and interpret sets of data in a similar manner. This has given rise to an over-use of tests of statistical significance in the interpretation of data arising from human populations. The extreme misuse is occasionally encountered where an author will equate "statistically significant" with "causually associated" and "not statistically significant" with "not associated". This issue will be discussed in a later section.

B. Human Populations

Data on human populations usually are not assembled in experimental settings, although there are exceptions. If one wishes to determine whether coal tar is carcinogenic to persons who work with it, an investigator does not gather a group of persons, randomly assign coal tar exposure to half of the group, and follow them to measure the rate of skin cancer. This would be neither ethical nor practical. Rather, one may measure the percentage of exposure to coal tar of persons with and without skin cancer, or may measure the rate of development of skin cancer in persons with and without exposure to coal tar.

However, an experiment on a human population is done in a setting analagous to that used with animal populations. Two other settings are common in collecting data on human health — the clinical and the epidemiologic.

1. The Clinical Setting

The practicing physician works primarily with persons who are ill. The primary impetus of a physician is to cure illness and relieve suffering. A secondary impetus is to prevent the occurrence of disease. Less emphasis is placed on the search for the causes of diseases.

Because of the nature of the clinical setting, data assembled by practicing physicians may be subject to misinterpretation. In the context of the cure of disease, a physician knows only whether a patient gets better. Many diseases are self-limiting and a person with the disease may get better irrespective of any treatment. If such a person sees a physician and is treated, it obviously is not possible to determine whether the treatment caused the cure of the disease.

Similar difficulties are present in the clinical evaluation of the causes of disease. The medical literature contains many "case reports" in which a physician reports her experiences with an unusual constellation of exposure and disease. For example, when oral contraceptives were first being used, there was a report of women taking oral contraceptives who developed high blood pressure.[1] It was not possible on the basis of such information to determine whether this represented an unusual occurrence, since it was likely this group of patients was selected from the physician's practice because of the joint occurrence of oral contraceptive use and hypertension.

The clinical setting, therefore, does not lend itself to providing definitive data on the association between disease and its causes, preventives, or cures. However, important information has been obtained in the clinical context. The clinician is usually the first person to see the patient with the first symptoms of a disease. As a result, the physician is closer in time to the etiologic event than is the epidemiologist. The clinician may have access to information that may not be obtainable by the epidemiologist. Because of this, the information entered by a clinician onto the medical record is vital to any later conduct of formal epidemiologic studies.

In the context of acute illnesses resulting from acute exposures, a clinician is the person most likely to detect the association. No formal study was needed to detect an association between the inhalation of SO_2 and acute bronchospasm. In fact no clinician need be present to make the connection. Simply stepping into an atmosphere containing SO_2 is sufficient to detect the etiologic association. Other causal associations are less apparent. However, it was an observant clinician who first recognized that working in a vinyl chloride polymerization plant led to the development of angiosarcoma of the liver many years later.[2]

2. The Epidemiologic Setting

In contrast to a clinician, whose main role is to cure disease, an epidemiologist is motivated to find the cause of disease. The epidemiologist, therefore, needs to collect data on exposures as well as diseases. Further, the epidemiologist has a fundamental concern with comparisons: she routinely compares the rate of illness in an exposed group to the rate in an unexposed group or compares the percentage of exposure in a diseased group to the percentage in a nondiseased group. This concern with comparability extends beyond the analysis of data. The collection of data also must be done in a comparable manner; for example, in comparing the rate of development of disease in a group of workers exposed to asbestos, equal care must be taken in following a comparison group of workers not exposed to asbestos.

This concern of epidemiologists with comparability cannot be overemphasized. The primary concern of the clinician is to cure the patient. If by prescribing penicillin to all persons with sore throats the patients get better, the clinician is relatively unconcerned whether the penicillin, in fact, cured the disease. The clinician in daily practice does not routinely compare the rate of cure of sore throat in patients treated with penicillin to the rate of cure in patients not treated. The clinician wishes to maximize the probability of cure, and if in her experience patients treated with penicillin tend to get better, she will continue to prescribe penicillin.

An experimentalist also has less active concern for comparability. Because of the ability to assign an exposure at random, there is much built-in comparability in experimental settings. An experimentalist has the same need for comparability between study groups as does an epidemiologist, but the effort needed to approach comparability is much less.

What is the source of the epidemiologist's striving for comparability? It lies in the largely unknown factors that lead to the development of disease. In an experiment one can essentially assure equal distribution of these unknown factors between exposed and control groups through randomization. In the natural setting of an epidemiologist, however, no such control is possible. Epidemiologists, therefore, seek to exert as much control as possible over which data are collected and the way the data are collected and analyzed. Central to this control is the assurance that comparable methods were used in collecting data from the two or more groups being compared.

Two features, therefore, characterize epidemiologic data:

1. The data derive from nonexperimental settings; as a result there is a basic noncomparability in groups of people with and without specific characteristics.
2. Because of this basic noncomparability of populations, there is a need to collect data in a comparable manner.

It may seem that if epidemiologic data derive from noncomparable groups, there is little value in worrying about comparability in assembling that data. On occasion, this is the case and no amount of epidemiologic expertise can help in evaluating a postulated association between exposure and disease. More usually, however, information may be collected on factors that are associated with the disease being evaluated.

Epidemiologic methods have been developed to assess the comparability of study groups by evaluating the interrelationships of these factors.

3. The Experimental Setting

As in animal populations, experiments may be done in human populations. Whereas in animal populations one can do experiments seeking the cause, prevention, or cure of disease, in human populations, experiments are done mainly to seek preventives or cures. Clearly, knowingly causing illness in humans raises serious ethical questions.

The basic methodology of an experiment in a human population is the same as that in an animal population. Exposure or nonexposure to an agent is solely determined by the investigator; random assignment of the agent assures comparability over the long run.

However, the conduct of an experiment in humans has important differences from the conduct in animals. There is far more variation within a human population than within an animal population. Therefore, even though random assignment to exposure is possible, in a given experiment chance may lead to a basic noncomparability of study and control group. Further, once the initial assignment is made, the investigator has much less control over humans than over animals. Even though there may be comparability between two study groups at the beginning of an experiment on humans, as the experiment progresses, noncomparability may develop.

III. EXAMPLES OF DATA

There are three basic questions that may be asked about the occurrence of disease in human populations:

1. Does an agent cause disease?
2. Does an agent prevent disease?
3. Does an agent cure disease?

Most medical research has as its goal the desire to answer one of these questions. The data resulting from investigations of one of these questions usually are assembled under differing conditions, but the numbers that result may usually be presented in the form of a fourfold table.

A. Causal Agents

1. The Clinical Setting

Suspicions from clinicians that an agent may be responsible for a disease frequently take the form of "case reports". A clinician notices what appears to be an unusual constellation of exposure and disease. A letter to the editor of a medical journal or a brief report follows.

Such reports frequently are faulted because "there is no control group". The lack of a control group is especially common in case-reports dealing with drugs taken during pregnancy. Consider the following case-reports:

1. Mothers of children with phocomelia (absent arms and legs) took thalidomide during pregnancy.[3]
2. Mothers of children with cleft palate took phenytoin during pregnancy.[4]
3. Mothers of chidren with malformations took aspirin during pregnancy.[5]

In each of these reports the possibility is raised that the drug taken during pregnancy was responsible for the malformation in the child. In the case of thalidomide and phocomelia, the assertion has great credibility since phocomelia is a very uncommon birth defect. However, cleft palate is a rather common malformation. The simple co-occurrence of phenytoin therapy and cleft palate does not necessarily reflect a causal association. Further, phenytoin is a specific drug used to treat a specific disease (epilepsy). How can the independent effects of epilepsy and phenytoin be evaluated? Aspirin on the other hand is a very common drug, usually taken for minor medical problems. If it affects the fetus adversely, even in a relatively low percentage of pregnancies, the implications would be great on public health.

2. The Epidemiologic Setting

After a causal association is postulated by a clinician in a case report, a number of similar case reports usually follow. Also, an epidemiologist becomes interested in the association and designs a study to collect some data. Ideally, the epidemiologist functions as a disinterested scientist and seeks to conduct her study in a neutral manner. On occasion, however, the epidemiologist starts a study either to prove the hypothesis or to show the inadequacy of the clinical method. Data resulting from one of these situations have the same appearance as data resulting from another. Only by reading the words of the author can an impression be gained as to the prior biases of the author. Even the words, of course, do not tell the whole story.

Essentially no epidemiologic studies followed the report of an association between thalidomide and phocomelia. The disease was extremely rare before the drug was marketed and extremely rare in children born to women who did not take the drug. No elaborate data analysis was needed to reveal the association. No careful consideration of the nature of the data was needed to interpret the nature of the association. It became obvious in a relatively short period of time that thalidomide caused phocomelia. The drug was removed from the market and the disease abated.

Several epidemiologic studies have been done to assess the postulated association between phenytoin and congenital malformations. In one report, data from two studies were presented (Table 2.2).[6]

In each study, an association between epilepsy and malformation is seen. In study one, the rate of malformation is almost two times higher in children of epileptics than in children of nonepileptics. In study two, the percentage of epileptic mothers who used phenytoin is four times higher in children with malformations than in those without.

However, the basic question is: "Does phenytoin ingestion during pregnancy cause a cleft palate in the fetus?" This question could not be addressed in study two, since no information was available on women who had epilepsy but who did not use phenytoin during pregnancy. In study one, this information was available (Table 2.3). In these data, within epileptic women, a negative association is seen between phenytoin use and a malformation in the offspring. Only 1 of the 21 malformations in the children born to the phenytoin-using women was a cleft palate.

These data from the epidemiologic setting were mainly collected prior to any suspicion that phenytoin caused any malformation. Thus there was comparability in the collection methods from users and nonusers or between malformed and normal children. However, a basic noncomparability remains in that phenytoin users are all epileptic while nonusers are mainly nonepileptic. Even when one limits the analysis to women with epilepsy, phenytoin users and nonusers probably differ in other ways. Therefore, while the data in Table 2.3 indicate no positive association between phenytoin and malformations, they do not necessarily convey absolute truth.

With respect to aspirin and malformation, in an epidemiologic study based on the

Table 2.2
RELATIONSHIP BETWEEN
MATERNAL EPILEPSY AND
CONGENITAL MALFORMATIONS
IN THE OFFSPRING IN TWO
STUDIES

Study 1

| Epilepsy | Malformation | | | Rate |
	Yes	No	Total	
Yes	32	273	305	10.5/100
No	3216	46,761	49,977	6.4/100
Total	3248	47,034	50,282	6.5/100

Study 2

| Epilepsy and phenytoin | Malformation | |
	Yes	No
Yes	8	2
No	2776	2782
Total	2784	2784
Percentage	0.29	0.07

Table 2.3
RELATIONSHIP BETWEEN MATERNAL
PHENYTOIN USE IN EPILEPTIC WOMEN
AND CONGENITAL MALFORMATIONS IN
THE OFFSPRING

| Phenytoin use in epileptic women | Malformation | | | Rate |
	Yes	No	Total	
Yes	21	187	208	10/100
No	11	86	97	11/100
Total	32	273	305	

same population as the phenytoin study one, no association between aspirin and malformations was seen.[7] In this context, however, there are different concerns. Because aspirin is so readily available and commonly used, there is concern that there is little reliability as to information concerning its use. Women who use aspirin may forget to report it while those who did not use it during pregnancy may incorrectly report having used it. If this were the case, a real association between aspirin and malformations may not be seen in the data. Those who are called "users" are in reality a mixture of users and nonusers. Likewise, those called "nonusers" include some users. The data

Table 2.4
RELATIONSHIP BETWEEN
MATERNAL PHENYTOIN AND
CONGENITAL CLEFT PALATE
IN THE OFFSPRING IN MICE

	Cleft palate			
Phenytoin	Yes	No	Total	Rate
Yes	11	48	59	19/100
No	0	61	61	0/100
Total	11	109	120	

data do not efficiently contain information on the association between aspirin use and malformation.

3. The Experimental Setting

There are essentially no data in humans from the experimental setting relating to drugs taken during pregnancy as possible causes of malformation. Clearly, if there is a strong suspicion such as with thalidomide, such a study would not be ethical. However, drugs such as phenytoin and aspirin continue to be used in pregnancy and continue to be useful. An experimental study of phenytoin use in epileptics probably could be done, provided that alternate means of controlling a woman's epilepsy were guaranteed. Such a study probably is the only way to collect definitive data on the interrelationships between epilepsy, phenytoin, and malformations.

An experimental evaluation of the relationship between aspirin taken in pregnancy and malformations in the offspring would be considerably more difficult. The assembly of a cooperative study population would be hard to do; the use of aspirin by those assigned to the nonuser group could not be easily monitored; the use of aspirin by those assigned to the user group could not be guaranteed. If a positive association were seen in such an experiment, it probably would be more likely to be believed than if no association were seen.

There are experimental data on animals on the association between phenytoin and cleft palate. In one study, injections of various doses of phenytoin were given to some mice and injections of a presumably harmless salt solution were given to others. The data are presented in Table 2.4.[8] Clearly, these data strongly suggest that this dose of phenytoin causes cleft palate in mice. However, the dose used is much greater than that in humans. Also, there is difficulty in relating data from mice to data from humans.

B. Preventive Agents
1. The Clinical Setting

Case-reports suggesting that a substance may be useful in the prevention of disease are less frequent than in the context of the cause of disease. This is because clinicians see patients with (caused) disease, not persons with (prevented) no disease. However, through clinical knowledge of the way drugs work, there may be hypotheses put forth relating to disease prevention.

Aspirin tends to prevent the aggregation of blood platelets and therefore to slow the coagulation of blood. Based on this fact, it was suggested that persons over the age of 40 take one aspirin a day to prevent heart attacks.[9] It was felt that little harm would

Table 2.5
RELATIONSHIP BETWEEN
ASPIRIN USAGE AND HEART
ATTACKS IN A GROUP OF
HOSPITALIZED PERSONS

	Heart attack	
Aspirin use	Yes	No
Yes	3	188
No	322	3619
Total	325	3807
Percentage	0.9	4.9

come from such a procedure, and the possibility of disease prevention was real. The only data used in this suggestion derived from the test tube.

2. The Epidemiologic Setting

At about the same time as the above suggestion was made, a study was underway in which data were collected on drug usage in hospitalized persons with a variety of diagnoses.[10] Included in the data was information on aspirin use among persons with and without heart attacks (Table 2.5). In these data a negative association between aspirin and heart attack is seen. This is consistent with the hypothesis that aspirin prevents heart attacks.

What interpretation of these data is to be made? Does one recommend that all persons should start taking aspirin so as to prevent heart attacks? Does one conclude that the investigators either through design or error caused these data to result? Or does one seek differences between persons with and without heart disease to explain the association? Clearly, the data by themselves do not prescribe which action to take.

3. The Experimental Setting

Whereas in the study of the cause of disease, experiments on human populations have limited utility, in the study of the prevention (or of the cure) of disease, experiments are naturally suited. One can select a population, randomly assign the potential preventive agent to one half and some other treatment to the other half, and follow the two groups to get data on the occurrence of disease. Naturally, the disease to be prevented must be expected to occur relatively soon after the start of the experiment.

The main use of experiments in the prevention of disease has been in evaluating immunization for the prevention of an infectious disease. In 1951, a report was published on the prevention of whooping cough. Children aged 6 to 18 months were randomly divided into two groups. One group was treated with influenza vaccine. After roughly 3 years of follow-up, the data in Table 2.6 were available.[11] Whether one looks at the attack rate or the incidence rate, it is clear that the rate of whooping cough was lower in the vaccinated than in the nonvaccinated children. Since the assignment to treatment was random, and since those treated did not know whether they had received whooping cough or influenza vaccine, the belief that whooping cough was prevented by the vaccine is strong.

Contrast this study with an experiment designed to collect data on the association between aspirin and mortality. Men who had had one heart attack were divided at

Table 2.6

RELATIONSHIP BETWEEN INNOCULATION WITH
WHOOPING COUGH VACCINE AND WHOOPING COUGH IN A
POPULATION OF SCHOOL CHILDREN

Whooping cough vaccine	Whooping cough			Rate A[a]	Rate B[b]
	Yes	No	Total		
Yes	149	3652	3801	39/1000	1.5/1000/month
No	687	3070	3757	180/1000	6.7/1000/month
Total	836	6722	7558	110/1000	4.1/1000/month

[a] "Attack rate" — # cases/1000 children.
[b] "Incidence rate" — # cases/1000 children/month.

Table 2.7

RELATIONSHIP BETWEEN
ASPIRIN USAGE AND DEATH
IN A CLINICAL TRIAL

Aspirin	Death			Rate
	Yes	No	Total	
Yes	47	519	566	8.3/1000
No	61	499	560	10.9/100
Total	108	1018	1126	

random into two groups: one group was given pills containing aspirin and the second was given pills containing a placebo (an inert substance). After one year of the experiment, the data seen in Table 2.7 were presented.[12] As in the epidemiologic study discussed above, aspirin appeared to have a beneficial effect. However, the magnitude of the effect was quite small. In the whooping cough study, the ratio of the two attack rates was $39 \div 180 = 0.22$. In the aspirin study, the ratio of the two attack rates was $8.3 \div 10.9 = 0.76$. Further, the number of persons under study in the whooping cough study was almost seven times that in the aspirin study. Therefore, there was greater stability in the data. That is, it would seem less likely that chance could have produced the results in the whooping cough study than in the aspirin study.

C. Curative Agents

1. The Clinical Setting

Probably no area of clinical medicine is more subject to controversy than is the consideration of cures of disease. From the beginning of medicine, physicians have found cures that with the passage of time have proven to be useless. This is true in the medical treatment of disease as well as in the surgical treatment. The basic motivation of a physician is to find ways of curing disease and to use those ways on as many patients as possible as soon as possible. This is humanitarian. However, the humanitarian needs of society must be balanced by its scientific needs, which are no less necessary. False cures or cures that do more harm than good are in the long run damaging to the patient.

Peptic ulcer is a common chronic disease. Persons with an ulcer may have repeated

Table 2.8
DATA FROM THE
CLINICAL SETTING ON
GASTRIC "FREEZING"
AND RELIEF OF PAIN

Stomach cooled	Pain relieved		
	Yes	No	Total
Yes	19	0	19
No	0	0	0
Total	19	0	19

Table 2.9
DATA FROM THE CLINICAL
SETTING ON CORONARY
ARTERY BYPASS SURGERY
AND ALLEVIATION OF
PAIN

Treated	Pain lessened		
	Yes	No	Total
Yes	77	25	102
No	0	0	0
Total	77	25	102

attacks of pain and bleeding. It is thought that an excess secretion of hydrochloric acid by the stomach may be responsible for the development of an ulcer in the duodenum. Therefore, if acid secretion can be reduced, the symptoms of an ulcer might abate.

One attempt to relieve the symptoms of peptic ulcer was gastric "freezing".[13] A balloon connected to a tube was passed into the stomach and a coolant at $-10°C$ was passed through the balloon. This resulted in a reduction in stomach secretion of acid. With respect to symptomatic relief the data were as shown in Table 2.8. Clearly, on clinical grounds, the treatment appeared to be of value.

Similar data were obtained from a clinical report of coronary artery bypass surgery. This is a procedure done for persons who have severe chest pain because of diminished blood flow to the heart. A vein graft is connected from the aorta to the artery supplying the heart, bypassing the occluded portion of the coronary artery. In one clinical report of such surgery, the results were as shown in Table 2.9.[14] Again, the treatment led to improvement of the patient's symptoms.

A third clinical study describes the treatment with L-DOPA of persons with Parkinson's disease. This is a potentially debilitating disease because of the progressive occurrence of involuntary movements of the hands coupled with a general loss in voluntary movement. On metabolic grounds, it was felt that the drug L-DOPA might relieve the symptoms of Parkinsonism. In an early clinical study, L-DOPA indeed seemed to be of value (Table 2.10).[15]

In each of these examples from the clinical setting, initial reports concerning a new treatment were promising. Clearly, however, one cannot judge whether the treatment itself led to the improvement or whether there was another reason. The disease may have abated spontaneously or simply being treated with something may have led to the reduction in symptoms. The data presented are insufficient to recommend that these treatments enter general medical practice.

2. The Epidemiologic Setting

Epidemiologic studies are limited in providing data relating to the efficacy of disease treatments. It is not difficult to accumulate data on the rate of cure of persons treated with a substance or procedure and compare this to the rate of persons treated with another therapy or of persons not treated.[16] This is quite similar to comparing rates of disease in persons exposed or not exposed to some agent.

However, the situations are not analogous. There tends to be an association between the severity of disease and the treatment used. Therefore, in looking at the rate of cure it is difficult to disentangle the treatment effect from the disease effect. Consider, for

Table 2.10
DATA FROM THE CLINICAL
SETTING ON L-DOPA
TREATMENT AND
ALLEVIATION OF SYMPTOMS
OF PARKINSON'S DISEASE

Treated	Symptoms reduced		
	Yes	No	Total
Yes	28	0	28
No	0	0	0
Total	28	0	28

Table 2.11
DATA FROM THE EXPERIMENTAL
SETTING ON THE RELATIONSHIP
BETWEEN GASTRIC "FREEZING"
AND CURED PEPTIC ULCER

"Freeze"	"Cured" at 24 months			"Cure" rate
	Yes	No	Total	
Yes	34	35	69	49/100
No	38	30	68	56/100
Total	72	65	137	

example, diabetes. Mild diabetes is treated with diet only, moderate diabetes is treated with oral medication, and severe diabetes is treated with insulin. If one compares the rate of cure in insulin-treated diabetics to the rate in diet-treated diabetics, it is not possible to determine if any differences seen in improvement of health are associated with the treatment or with the disease.

This argument, however, does not hold true in all situations, and epidemiologic comparisons can be made. However, since there is an alternative that is clearly preferable — the clinical trial — such comparisons are infrequent.

3. The Experimental Setting

Experiments on human populations in evaluating the potential value of a treatment of disease are called clinical trials. Here the word clinical is used because the experiment is conducted in a medical setting. Clinical trials are of great importance in assessing whether newly-developed treatments of disease are of value.

Consider gastric freezing. In 1969, a report describing a clinical trial of gastric freezing was published.[17] In this trial 137 persons with duodenal ulcer were enrolled. After being informed of the nature of the study, 69 received the "freeze" treatment described above; 68 had the balloon placed in the stomach, but the cold liquid circulated only to the esophagus. Thus there was no cooling of the acid-producing cells of the stomach. The two groups were followed for 24 months or until severe ulcer symptoms recurred. The following data were obtained (Table 2.11). Clearly, there was no evidence that gastric freezing cured peptic ulcer. If anything, the freeze patients had a lower cure rate than those whose stomachs were not frozen.

Similar results were obtained in a clinical trial of coronary artery bypass surgery.[18] A group of persons with coronary artery disease were enrolled and told about the proposed study. Those who agreed to participate were assigned either to medical or to surgical therapy. Medical therapy involved the usual medical practice, primarily with drugs. Surgical therapy was coronary artery bypass surgery, as described above. At 3 years, 87% of the medical group and 88% of the surgical group were alive. This is very weak support for the contention that surgical therapy for this disease is superior to medical therapy, at least with respect to subsequent mortality.

On the other hand, there is little question that L-DOPA relieves the symptoms of Parkinson's disease. Patients who were incapacitated because of their symptoms were returned to near-normal life. However, not all persons are helped. Also, there is always the possibility of adverse long-term effects. Because Parkinson's disease is an illness that occurs in older persons, and because the symptoms are so debilitating, any long-term effects of L-DOPA must be serious to counter-balance its beneficial effects.

IV. MEASURES OF DISEASE FREQUENCY

A. Types

In the examples presented above, data have been presented in the form of a fourfold table. The numbers are summarized either as rates of disease or percentages of exposure. By so summarizing the data, comparisons can be made of two or more groups.

The basic measure underlying epidemiologic data is the *rate:* the quantity or degree of a thing measured per unit of something else. The *thing* is number of cases of a disease; the *something else* is number of persons in the group within whom the disease occurred. In epidemiologic studies, the basic comparison is the ratio between disease rates in two populations.

There are three basic types of disease rates that concern a person interested in occupational epidemiology. One is the *incidence rate:* the number of cases of disease per unit population per unit time. For example, if of 1000 workers who enter employment 10 develop arthritis in the next 10 years, the incidence rate is 10/1000/10 years or 1/1000/year. Incidence rate, then, refers to the development of new disease over some period of time. A *mortality rate* is an example of an incidence rate, where the new disease is death. For example, the average annual mortality rate of U.S. white males is approximately 10/1000/year.

The *prevalence rate* measures numbers of existing diseases in a population; its unit is cases per unit population. For example, in an employed population of average age 55, 5% of the persons may have diabetes: the prevalence rate is 5/100. The prevalence rate is useful in studies where comparisons are made between the presence of disease in two or more groups.

Whereas interpretation of an incidence rate is relatively straightforward, there are several factors that influence the prevalence rate. In general, if the incidence rate (I) increases, the prevalence rate (P) increases. If the duration (D) of a disease increases, the prevalence rate increases. If the "cure rate" (C) of a disease increases, the prevalence rate decreases. If the mortality rate (M) of a disease increases, the prevalence rate decreases. This may be expressed as:

$$P = (I - C - M) D \qquad\qquad (2.1)$$

The units of the above equation are: P — cases/unit population; I, C, M — cases/unit population/unit time; and D — time.

A third type of rate has the concept of incidence but the units of prevalence: the *attack rate.* An attack rate is the number of cases of disease that develop in a population during some fixed time period; the unit is cases per population. Attack rates are used in infectious disease epidemiology where an acute disease occurs in a population and then abates. The number of persons in the population is the same at the end as at the beginning of the epidemic. The attack rate is the number who become ill divided by the total number in the population. Another use of an attack rate is in experiments; if the time of follow-up is the same for the exposed and control groups, the attack rate may be used to measure the rate of disease occurrence in each group.

As indicated, a mortality rate is an example of an incidence rate. A birth rate is also an incidence rate: births/1000 population/year. However, a birth-defect rate is a prevalence rate: children with a defect divided by total children born. This measure is frequently misused.

B. Comparisons

Rates of different types should not be compared. It is erroneous to compare the incidence rate of peptic ulcer in one population to the prevalence rate in a second. The only way a prevalence rate can be related to an incidence rate is in the computation of the duration of a disease. However, rates of similar types are to be compared. Such comparisons are central to analysis of epidemiologic data.

1. Rate Ratio (Risk Ratio, Relative Risk)

The fourfold table (Table 2.1) has within it rates of disease. If "a" is number of persons with disease in an exposed group of size "a + b", then $a/(a + b)$ is the prevalence rate. Likewise, $c/(c + d)$ is the prevalence rate in the nonexposed group. In order to compare these rates, one simple method is to divide one by the other. This is the "rate ratio": $a/(a + b) \div c/(c + d)$.

$$RR = R_e \div R_o \qquad (2.2)$$

In words, Formula 2.2 states that the rate ratio equals the rate of disease in the exposed (R_e) divided by the rate in the nonexposed (R_o).

This is the most basic comparison in epidemiology and indeed in everyday life. Instead of exposure being yes and no, it could be Store A and Store B. If the cost of steak is $2.00/lb in Store A and $1.50/lb in Store B, the ratio of these two costs (rates) is $2.00/$1.50 = 1.33.

The basic idea of the fourfold table also underlies the comparisons of incidence rates. In such an example, "a" and "c" represent the numbers of persons in the two groups who have developed a disease. The denominators are person-years rather than persons. Thus, if 10 cases of disease develop in 100 exposed persons followed for an average of 4 years, the incidence rate in the exposed would be 10/100/4 years or 10/400 person-years. In the nonexposed group the rate might be 6/100/3 years or 6/300 person-years. The rate ratio is $10/400 \div 6/300 = 1.25$. Note that an incidence rate of 10/400 person-years is the same as 10/400 persons/year or 10/100 persons/4 years.

2. Rate Difference (Risk Difference, Attributable Risk)

Just as the rate ratio is one rate divided by a second, the rate difference is one rate minus a second. In the case of the prevalence rate example, the rate difference is $a/(a + b) - c/(c + d)$.

$$RD = R_e - R_o \qquad (2.3)$$

In words, Formula 2.3 states that the rate difference (RD) equals the rate of disease in the exposed (R_e) minus the rate in the nonexposed (R_o). In the example of the cost of meat, the rate difference is $2.00/lb − $1.50/lb = $0.50/lb. In the example of incidence rates, the rate difference is 10/400 person-years − 6/300 person years = 2.5/100 − 2.0/100 = 0.5/100 person-years.

Note that the rate ratio has no units while the rate difference has the units of the rates being subtracted. The rate ratio provides a relative measure of the two rates while

Table 2.12

THE RELATIONSHIP BETWEEN CIGARETTE SMOKING AND LUNG CANCER AND ISCHEMIC HEART DISEASE

A.	Cigarette smoking			Rate of lung cancer
	Yes			140/100,000/year
	No			10/100,000/year
	Rate difference:	140 − 10	=	130/100,000/year
	Rate ratio:	140/10	=	14.0
B.	Cigarette smoking			Rate of ischemic heart disease
	Yes			669/100,000/year
	No			413/100,000/year
	Rate difference:	669 − 413	= 256/100,000/year	
	Rate ratio:	669/413	= 1.6	

the rate difference provides an absolute comparison. The rate ratio is more commonly used, because it gives the most intuitive comparison.

There is no necessary connection between the size of the rate ratio and the size of the rate difference. Consider the following examples (Table 2.12).[19] The rate ratio for lung cancer in smokers is much higher than that for ischemic heart disease; however, the rate difference is 50% lower.

This example illustrates the basic noncomparability of these two measures. The very high rate ratio for lung cancer in smokers argues for the causal nature of the association. The relatively low rate ratio for ischemic heart disease means that consideration must be given to other factors that may account for the association between cigarette smoking and ischemic heart disease. On the other hand, if it is true that cigarette smoking causes death from lung cancer and from ischemic heart disease, twice as many men die per year from cigarette-induced heart disease as from cigarette-induced lung cancer.

The basic reason for the apparently different impressions gained from the rate ratio and the rate difference is in the size of the rate in nonsmokers. Ischemic heart disease is over 40 times as common as lung cancer in nonsmokers. Therefore, even a relatively small increase in the rate will affect many more persons than will the relatively large increase in the rate of lung cancer.

V. SUMMARY

Data are numbers — nothing less and nothing more. Without knowledge of the source of the data and of the means by which the data were collected, no inferences can be made as to the meaning of the data.

However, all information is based on data. We have no other way of gaining knowledge. Therefore, data cannot be dismissed simply because they are numbers. In order to interpret data — in order to seek the significance of associations — it must first be recognized that data form the basis of human knowledge. Of equal importance, however, is the recognition that all data are imperfect, no matter what their source or how they were collected.

There are few absolutes. Few sets of data are worthless and few convey absolute truth. The task facing epidemiologists as well as all other persons is to decide how to judge the validity of data. The source of the data may not be ideal, but it may be the only source available. The data may have not been collected under absolutely correct circumstances, but the error introduced may be small. The analysis of the data may have been superficial, but further analyses may add little to the understanding of the meaning of any association seen.

The interpretation of the meaning of data must take into account all these considerations of data source, means of collection, and methods of analysis. This is largely a scientific process — one in which the judgment of one's peers is most important. However, decisions as to the utility of the data and the changes in behavior that may result from the information contained in the data must be based on an independent process that is largely political — one in which the data collector and indeed the scientific field must also be judged.

The role of an epidemiologist is to collect and analyze data as a disinterested observer. Only if this attitude is maintained can there be a hope that knowledge is gained as to true causal associations between exposure and disease in human populations. An epidemiologist may be motivated to conduct studies because of the belief that certain associations exist, but this belief must not affect the conduct of the study. Because epidemiologists are imperfect, and because the maintenance of disinterest cannot always be guaranteed, judgments to the meaning of the results of any study must be made by independent observers.

REFERENCES

1. Woods, J. W., Oral contraceptives and hypertension, *Lancet*, 2, 653, 1967.
2. Creech, J. L., Jr. and Johnson, M. N., Angiosarcoma of liver in the manufacture of polyvinyl chloride, *J. Occup. Med.*, 16, 150, 1974.
3. McBride, W. G., The teratogenic action of drugs, *Med. J. Aust.*, 2, 689, 1963.
4. Meadow, S. R., Anticonvulsant drugs and congenital abnormalities, *Lancet*, 2, 1296, 1968.
5. Richards, I. D. G., Congenital malformations and environmental influences in pregnancy, *Br. J. Prev. Soc. Med.*, 23, 218, 1969.
6. Shapiro, S., Slone, D., Hartz, S. C., Rosenberg, L., Siskind, V., Monson, R. R., Mitchell, A. A., Heinonen, O. P., Idänpään-Heikkilä, J., Härö, S., and Saxén, L., Anticonvulsants and parental epilepsy in the development of birth defects, *Lancet*, 1, 272, 1976.
7. Slone, S., Siskind, V., Heinonen, O. P., Monson, R. R., Kaufman, D. W., and Shapiro, S., Aspirin and congenital malformations, *Lancet*, 1, 1373, 1976.
8. Elshove, J., Cleft palate in the offspring of female mice treated with phenytoin, *Lancet*, 2, 1074, 1969.
9. Wood, L., Treatment of atheroslcerosis and thrombosis with aspirin, *Lancet*, 2, 532, 1972.
10. Boston Collaborative Drug Surveillance Program, Regular aspirin intake and acute myocardial infarction, *Br. Med. J.*, 1, 440, 1974.
11. Medical Research Council, The prevention of whooping-cough by vaccination, *Br. Med. J.*, 1, 1463, 1951.
12. Elwood, P. C., Cochrane, A. L., Burr, J. L., Sweetnam, P. M., Williams, G., Welshy, E., Hughes, S. J., and Renton, R., A randomized controlled trial of acetyl salicylic acid in the secondary prevention of mortality from myocardial infarction, *Br. Med. J.*, 1, 436, 1974.
13. Wangensteen, O. H., Peter, E. T., Bernstein, E. F., Walder, A. I., Sosin, H., and Madsen, A. J., Can physiological gastrectomy be achieved by gastric freezing? *Ann. Surg.*, 156, 579, 1962.
14. Alderman, E. L., Matlof, H. J., Wexler, L., Shumway, N. E., and Harrison, D. C., Results of direct coronary-artery surgery for the treatment of angina pectoris, *N. Engl. J. Med.*, 288, 535, 1973.
15. Cotzias, G. C., Papavasiliou, P. S., and Gellene, R., Modification of Parkinsonism — chronic treatment with L-DOPA, *N. Engl. J. Med.*, 280, 337, 1969.
16. Gehan, E. A. and Freireich, E. J., Non-randomized controls in cancer clinical trials, *N. Engl. J. Med.*, 290, 198, 1974.

17. Ruffin, J. M., Grizzle, J. E., Hightower, N. C., McHardy, G., Shull, H., and Kirsner, J. B., Gastric "freezing" in the treatment of duodenal ulcer, *N. Engl. J. Med.,* 281, 16, 1969.
18. Murphy, M. L., Hultgren, H. N., Detre, K., Thomsen, J., and Takaro, T., Treatment of chronic stable angina, *N. Engl. J. Med.,* 297, 621, 1977.
19. Doll, R. and Peto, R., Mortality in relation to smoking: 20 years' observations on male British doctors, *Br. Med. J.,* 2, 1525, 1976.

Chapter 3
THE COLLECTION OF EPIDEMIOLOGIC DATA

I. INTRODUCTION

In Chapter 2 the nature of data was discussed and examples were given of how data are used to show associations between exposures and diseases. In this chapter the methods used in epidemiology to obtain the data will be discussed. These methods are not unique to epidemiology, but are part of the general methodology of scientific inquiry. However, inasmuch as epidemiology is largely nonexperimental, there are different emphases than in the experimental sciences.

The main emphasis in the design and conduct of an epidemiologic study is *comparability.* In an experimental study it is straightforward to assemble groups of comparable subjects and to observe each group in a comparable manner. (This is true more for animals than for humans). But in a nonexperimental epidemiologic study, noncomparability is guaranteed from the beginning, and major efforts are needed in order to be able to demonstrate that any results have meaning in spite of this noncomparability.

A second concern in an epidemiologic study relates to the *selection of study groups.* Should one examine previously collected data? Should one assemble groups of exposed and nonexposed persons and follow them until disease occurs? Should one assemble groups of person with and without disease and interview them about past exposures? Should one collect information on exposure and disease simultaneously? Should one attempt to conduct an experiment to evaluate the association between exposure and disease?.

There are no standard answers to these questions in a given situation. Much depends upon the constraints of time, money, access to information and personal taste. Usually, once a question has been raised as to the possible effects of an exposure or the possible causes of a disease, a variety of studies are considered and carried out. In this chapter the design of such studies will be outlined.

II. TYPES OF STUDIES

Studies in epidemiology seek to find associations between exposure and disease (cause and effect). The main constraint of this relationship is that the exposure must occur before the disease. Graphically, this is presented in Figure 3.1.

The epidemiologist must select study groups on the basis of either a person's disease status or exposure status. Further, the epidemiologist may be at a number of points along the time axis when the study is conducted.

Any classification of types of epidemiologic studies is subject to criticism, just as is any glossary of epidemiologic terms. I find the following scheme to be useful:

1. Experimental
2. Nonexperimental
   a. Descriptive
   b. Analytic
      (1) Longitudinal
         (a) Cohort
            i. Prospective
            ii. Retrospective
         (b) Case-control
      (2) Cross-sectional

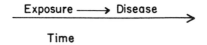

FIGURE 3.1.   The basic relationship in
epidemiology.

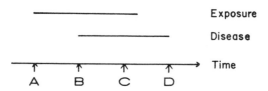

FIGURE 3.2.   Six basic study types in epidemiology.
1. Experimental: Investigator at time A assigns exposure. 2. Descriptive: Investigator measures exposure at
time A, or measures disease at time B (incidence), C
(prevalence), or D (mortality). 3. Prospective cohort:
Investigator at time A selects study groups on the basis
of exposure. 4. Retrospective cohort: Investigator at
time B, C, or D selects study groups on the basis of
exposure. 5. Case-control: Investigator at time B, C, or
D selects study groups on the basis of disease. 6. Cross-
sectional: Investigator at time C measures exposure and
disease simultaneously.

In an experimental study, the assignment of exposure to a study participant is under
the control of the investigator. In a nonexperimental study, the investigator has no
control over exposure.

In a descriptive study, either information is available on exposure and disease for
groups of persons only, or information is available for an individual only on exposure
or on disease. In an analytic study, information on exposure *and* disease is available
for each individual.

In a longitudinal study, the time sequence between the exposure and the disease can
be inferred. In a cross-sectional study, the data on exposure and disease relate to the
same point of time.

In a cohort study, individuals enter the study on the basis of exposure and nonexposure. In a case-control study, individuals enter the study on the basis of disease and
nondisease.

In a prospective cohort study, the disease has *not* occurred at the time the exposed
and nonexposed groups are defined. In a retrospective cohort study, the disease *has*
occurred at the time the exposed and nonexposed groups are defined.

Six basic study types are exemplified in Figure 3.2.

Each of these study types will be discussed later in this chapter. First, however, an
issue of importance in all studies — comparability of data — will be considered.

III. COMPARABILITY

If noncomparable criteria are used to select entrants into two groups of a study, the
data cannot be used to measure any postulated association between exposure and disease because of *selection bias*. If data are collected on two groups using noncomparable
methods, the data contain incorrect information as to exposure and disease because
of *observation bias*. If there are characteristics of persons that are associated both with

exposure and disease, the data relating exposure to disease may convey an appearance of association because of *confounding bias*.

Selection bias and observation bias result because of deficiencies in study design and data collection. These sources of bias are not inevitable, but are not always preventable. They must be considered in the design of a study and efforts must be made to minimize the effects of such bias.

Confounding bias is inevitable in all studies. In experimental studies, such bias tends to be minimized — but not necessarily controlled — because of random assignment of exposure. In nonexperimental studies, however, it is never possible to know all of the effects of confounding bias. All that is possible is to collect information on known or suspected confounding factors so as to be able to measure any bias introduced. Confounding bias does not result from any error of the investigator; it is a basic characteristic of existence.

A. Selection Bias

Selection bias occurs only in study design. For it to occur, the disease must have taken place at the time a person is enrolled into the study. Selection bias cannot be controlled; it must be prevented.

In an experiment, no selection bias is possible because the disease has not occurred at the time the exposure is assigned. Also, if two groups of persons — one exposed and one not exposed — are identified today and followed forward in time until disease occurs (prospective cohort study), no selection bias is possible.

Consider a study where a group of persons with disease is identified and a second group of controls is selected (a case-control study). Since at the time of entrance into the study group the disease has occurred, selection bias is possible. It results from the selective admission of exposed persons into the diseased group. (It may also result from the selective admission of exposed persons into the controls, of nonexposed persons into the cases, or of nonexposed persons into the controls). The central feature is that different criteria relating to exposure are used for entrance into the two groups.

An analogous situation exists when the initial study groups are exposed and nonexposed persons (a cohort study). However, selection bias may occur only in retrospective cohort studies — those where past records are used to define the study group and disease has already occurred when individuals are entered into the study. Selection bias results if there is noncomparable admission of diseased (or nondiseased) persons into the exposed (or nonexposed) group. Note that there must be a *difference* in the selection criteria between the two groups in order for bias to result. If there is an inaccurate definition of disease or of exposure that applies equally to the two groups, so-called "random misclassification" occurs (See Chapter 5).

Once selection bias has occurred, no amount of data manipulation can correct its effects. The two groups are forever noncomparable.

Selection bias can readily be prevented in retrospective cohort studies if knowledge of disease is masked in the selection of entrants. One uses only exposure criteria in defining exposed and nonexposed groups. Information on disease is collected only after the two study groups have been defined.

In case-control studies, selection bias can be prevented if knowledge of exposure is masked in selection of diseased and nondiseased groups. However, in contrast to cohort studies, such masking is not a simple matter. The criteria used in making a diagnosis on occasion include knowledge of exposure. Of even greater concern is the possibility that persons with certain symptoms are admitted to the hospital (and called diseased) if they have a certain exposure characteristic, but not admitted (and not diagnosed) if they do not have the exposure characteristic. Thus, in case-control studies, selection bias may not only be introduced by the investigator, but may be present without his knowledge.

For illnesses that are uniformly severe (heart attacks, appendicitis, acute cholecystitis), selection bias because of differential hospitalization is unlikely since all persons with the disease are admitted to the hospital. However, in diseases such as cancer where the symptoms of the disease develop slowly, selective hospitalization is likely. For example, if estrogen is suspected as being a cause of uterine cancer, women with abnormal vaginal bleeding who are taking estrogens may be admitted to the hospital in preference to those with bleeding who are not taking estrogen. Since some of the women who have bleeding also have cancer of the uterus, the percentage of estrogen use among those women will be artificially high. This fact will not be readily apparent from the data available on hospitalized patients.

Selection bias is usually discussed but rarely demonstrated. It may be offered as a theoretical objection to associations seen in hospital based case-control studies.[1] However, in a recent report measurements of selection bias have been made.[2]

B. Observation Bias (Information Bias)

In experimental or in cohort studies, observation bias results when information on disease outcome is obtained in a noncomparable manner from exposed and nonexposed groups. In case-control studies, observation bias results when information on exposure is obtained in a noncomparable manner from cases and controls.

An obvious way to prevent observation bias in an experiment or cohort study is not to know the exposure status of study individuals when information on disease is obtained. Any errors in measurement will be made equally in members of the exposed and nonexposed groups. Likewise, in a case-control study, no observation bias is possible if neither the patient nor the data collector know the diagnosis when information on exposure is collected. This characteristic of data collection is termed *blindness*.

Frequently, blindness is not possible in a case-control study. The patient knows his diagnosis or the interviewer knows which patients are cases and which are controls. To minimize observation bias in such a situation, *objectivity* is sought in obtaining information. Questions are asked that require objective answers (close-ended) rather than subjective answers (open-ended). While this does not prevent observation bias, it tends to minimize it.

Observation bias results because patients, epidemiologists, and data collectors are human. Patients, for the most part, are cooperative and wish to assist data collectors in every way possible. If the data collector explains in great detail the reasons a study is being done, the patient may give answers to help the data collector "prove" the association being evaluated. Data collectors may seek to please the epidemiologist by obtaining (biased) information that will help the epidemiologist write an interesting report. They may push harder in cases than in controls for positive answers to critical questions. Epidemiologists may have a pet theory on which data are being collected. In order to "prove" his theory, the epidemiologist may, through misguided enthusiasm, design the questionnaire and train data collectors in such a way so as to guarantee the desired result.

Underlying the prevention of observation bias is the need for all concerned with a study to be disinterested (impartial, unbiased). While it is important that scientific curiosity and enthusiasm lead an epidemiologist into areas of inquiry, once a study begins he must stand back from the reason for the study and conduct it without concern for the direction of the results. The only concern must be that the data collected reflect nature rather than the bias of the investigator.

For this reason, once an investigator has decided to study a postulated association ("test a hypothesis"), it is wise to set the hypothesis aside. The study should be designed so as to collect the information needed to evaluate the association, but additional information should also be collected. This will serve the dual purpose of enlarging the information collected as well as minimizing attention on the question being evaluated. To the extent that the study can be presented as a general evaluation of some exposure or of some disease, rather than the evaluation of the specific relationship between an exposure and a disease, the likelihood of observation bias is minimized.

This is not to say that everyone connected with a study should be kept in the dark as to its purpose. However, once an epidemiologist has decided to collect data, he will minimize observation bias by designing a broad, rather than a narrow, study. For example, in evaluating whether aspirin prevents heart attacks, the investigators designed a case-control study to collect data on all medications taken by persons with heart attacks and by controls.[3] In so doing, neither the interviewers nor the patients knew the specific reason for the study. Likewise, in a cohort study set up to evaluate the association between radiation exposure and breast cancer, information was collected on all cancers.[4]

C. Confounding Bias

Confounding bias is potentially and probably present in all data. It always must be considered as the possible explanation for any association seen in any data.

In evaluating an association between one variable (exposure) and a second (disease), confounding bias results when there exists a third variable that is a cause of the disease and also is associated with the exposure. Cigarette smoking is a cause of lung cancer. Cigarette smoking is associated with heavy alcohol drinking. If one looks at data on the relationship between heavy drinking and lung cancer, an association will be seen in that the rate of lung cancer in heavy drinkers is higher than the rate in nondrinkers. However, alcohol drinking probably does not cause lung cancer. The positive association between the two results from the confounding effects of cigarette smoking. If one looks at the association between alcohol and lung cancer in nonsmokers, no association is seen. If one looks at the association between alcohol and lung cancer in heavy smokers, no relationship is seen.

I am unaware of data illustrating the above example. Therefore, the data in Table 3.1 have been made up.

As can be seen in the table for all persons, the rate of lung cancer in alcohol users is 50% greater than that in nonusers. However, when one looks at the association within nonsmokers and smokers separately, there is essentially no association. This occurs because smoking is more common among alcohol users (60%) than nonusers (40%) *and* because lung cancer is more common among smokers than nonsmokers (90/1000 vs. 10/1000).

In order for a third variable to be confounding, it must be associated both with exposure and disease. If some variable is associated with disease but not with exposure, or vice versa, it cannot be confounding. Consider again alcohol, cigarette smoking, and lung cancer. If there is no association between alcohol and smoking, no confounding from smoking results even if it is a cause of lung cancer. This is illustrated in Table 3.2.

As can be seen in this example, cigarette smoking is associated with lung cancer but not with alcohol use. The rate ratio of 1.0 in the overall table is seen also in the smoking-specific tables. The same results would be seen if smoking were associated with alcohol use but not with lung cancer.

An understanding of this characteristic of confounding is essential in the design and analysis of epidemiologic studies. If a factor can be made or demonstrated to have no

Table 3.1
DERIVED DATA ILLUSTRATING
CONFOUNDING BY CIGARETTE
SMOKING IN EVALUATING THE
RELATIONSHIP BETWEEN
ALCOHOL USE AND LUNG CANCER

All persons

Alcohol user	Lung cancer		Total	Rate
	Yes	No		
Yes	60	940	1000	60/1000
No	40	960	1000	40/1000
Total	100	1900	2000	50/1000

Rate ratio = 60/40 = 1.5

Nonsmokers

Alcohol user	Lung cancer		Total	Rate
	Yes	No		
Yes	4	396	400	10/1000
No	6	594	600	10/1000
Total	10	990	1000	10/1000

Rate ratio = 10/10 = 1.0

Smokers

Alcohol user	Lung cancer		Total	Rate
	Yes	No		
Yes	56	544	600	93/1000
No	34	366	400	85/1000
Total	90	910	1000	90/1000

Rate ratio = 93/85 = 1.1

association with exposure, or with disease, that factor cannot be confounding. Recognition of the need of a confounding factor to be associated both with exposure and with disease is central to the prevention or control of confounding.

There are procedures designed to minimize confounding bias both in the design of the study and during data analysis. They include randomization, matching, and stratification. Randomization is a feature of study design, matching may be done either in the design of a study or in the analysis of data, and stratification (or standardization) is a feature of data analysis.

1. Randomization
Randomization is possible only in the experimental setting. It means the random assignment of exposure to one group and the random assignment of nonexposure to

Table 3.2
DERIVED DATA ILLUSTRATING NO
CONFOUNDING BY CIGARETTE
SMOKING IN EVALUATING THE
ASSOCIATION BETWEEN ALCOHOL
USE AND LUNG CANCER

All persons

Alcohol user	Lung cancer			Rate
	Yes	No	Total	
Yes	50	950	1000	50/1000
No	50	950	1000	50/1000
Total	100	1900	2000	50/1000

Rate ratio = 50/50 = 1.0

Nonsmokers

Alcohol user	Lung cancer			Rate
	Yes	No	Total	
Yes	5	495	500	10/1000
No	5	495	500	10/1000
Total	10	990	1000	10/1000

Rate ratio = 10/10 = 1.0

Smokers

Alcohol user	Lung cancer			Rate
	Yes	No	Total	
Yes	45	455	500	90/1000
No	45	455	500	90/1000
Total	90	910	1000	90/1000

Rate ratio = 90/90 = 1.0

the second group. Random essentially means by chance; each individual has an equal probability of being assigned to the exposed or to the nonexposed group.

Because of this random assignment of exposure in an experiment, all factors, confounding or not, tend to be distributed equally between exposed and nonexposed groups. Therefore, there tends to be no association between exposure and any factor. Factors associated with the development of the disease (causes of the disease) tend to be equally represented in the study groups and therefore tend not to be confounding.

Note that randomization does not guarantee comparability of confounding factors. In any given experimental study a cause of the disease (other than the exposure) may by chance occur more frequently among the exposed group than among the nonexposed group. This factor therefore will be confounding. However, it is likely that in the long run such factors will tend to distribute equally between exposed and nonexposed groups. Therefore, if experiments are repeated, and similar associations between exposure and disease are seen, confounding is an unlikely explanation.

While randomization does not guarantee that confounding is not present from any single factor in any given experiment, it has the powerful feature that all potential confounding factors — both recognized and unrecognized — tend to be randomly distributed. In nonexperimental studies, confounding can be evaluated only for causes of disease on which information is available. Since most causes of disease are not known, most potential confounding cannot be evaluated.

2. Matching

Matching is the usual method used in the design of nonexperimental studies to prevent confounding. (Matching may also be done in experiments). In a cohort study, matching means selecting individuals such that there is an equal frequency of persons with the potential confounding factor among exposed and nonexposed groups. In a case-control study, matching leads to an equal frequency of the potential confounding factor among diseased and nondiseased groups. Matching may be either *pair-wise* (for each exposed person with the factor, a nonexposed person with the factor is selected, etc.), or *frequency* (the percentage of persons with the factor is the same in the exposed and nonexposed groups, etc.).

Matching guarantees comparability between two groups, but only for the factor(s) matched. If a group of alcohol drinkers contains the same percentage of smokers as does a comparison group of nondrinkers, no confounding from smoking is possible. Confounding is still possible from all other factors.

If only one factor is to be controlled by matching, few problems exist. However, as more and more potential confounding factors are to be controlled by matching, extreme difficulties arise. If one wishes to do pair-wise matching of five dichotomous (yes/no) factors, there are 32 (2^5) possible conditions to be considered. It rapidly becomes difficult to find cases and controls who "match" each other on all characteristics. In frequency matching these constraints are relaxed, but the two groups do not have the same degree of comparability.

A characteristic of matching is that if a factor is matched, that factor cannot be evaluated in the study. If, in a case-control study, one matches cases to controls on age, no information on the association between age and the disease will be obtained. It is even not known whether the age could have been confounding, since no association with the disease has been guaranteed by the matching.

Partly because of the practical difficulties imposed by matching in the data collection phase of a study, partly because of the loss of potential information, partly because a suitable alternate is available, and partly because it may not be necessary, I tend to avoid matching in collecting data. By so doing, "over-matching" is avoided.

Over-matching is a problem in case-control studies. A confounding factor is one that is associated with exposure and independently is a cause of the disease. Some factors, however, are part of the causal chain leading from the exposure to the disease. For example, if salt in the diet leads to high blood pressure leads to strokes, it would not be proper to match on high blood pressure in evaluating an association between salt and stroke.

While such situations may appear to be obvious, a current controversy has arisen because of over-matching. In 1974, an association was reported between estrogen use and endometrial cancer. The data are presented in Table 3.3.[5] A clear cut association

Table 3.3 RELATIONSHIP BETWEEN ESTROGEN USE AND ENDOMETRIAL CANCER IN A CASE-CONTROL STUDY[5]					Table 3.4 RELATIONSHIP BETWEEN ESTROGEN USE AND ENDOMETRIAL CANCER IN A CASE-CONTROL STUDY[6]		
	Endometrial cancer					Endometrial cancer	
Estrogen use	Yes	No			Estrogen use	Yes	No
Yes	54	29			Yes	44	23
No	40	159			No	105	126
Total	94	188			Total	149	149
% Exposure	57	15			% Exposure	30	15

between estrogen use and endometrial cancer was apparent. However, it was argued that women who use estrogens have more uterine bleeding and therefore are subject to more diagnostic tests and therefore are more likely to have uterine cancer diagnosed. Therefore, a case-control study was done where a correlate of uterine bleeding was matched upon. The following data resulted (Table 3.4).[6]

The authors matched on having had a diagnostic test that is used on women with uterine bleeding. By so doing they essentially matched on uterine bleeding (over-matched), which is associated with estrogen use. However, in spite of the probable over-matching, an association was seen.

Based on the above, there are several criteria that should be met if one is to consider designing a "matched" study:

1. There should be no interest in evaluating the association between the disease and the factor to be matched.
2. There should be a reasonable likelihood that, if matching is not done, the factor will be confounding.
3. There should be a reasonable likelihood that the amount of confounding introduced is more than trivial.
4. There should be no possibility that the factor is part of the causal pathway linking the exposure and disease under study.

If there is a question about any of the above criteria, matching should not be done. Rather, any potential confounding introduced by the presence of the factor can be controlled in the analysis.

The term "matching" is frequently used to describe a feature of study design more related to convenience than to the control of confounding. If, in a case-control study, the investigator selects cases and controls from some large pool of potential participants, the case-control ratio should not be grossly disparate. Usual case-control ratios range from 1:1 to 1:4. Frequently, it is convenient to select one to four controls for each case. Such controls may be described as being "matched", in that they were selected at the same time, were in the same hospital, came from the same set of records, etc. as the cases. This "matching" is mainly for the convenience of the investigator rather than for the control of confounding. The variables matched upon are usually not important sources of confounding. Similar considerations hold true in a cohort study.

IV. EXAMPLES OF EPIDEMIOLOGIC STUDIES

A. Experimental Studies

In previous pages I have discussed the nature of data derived from experimental studies and have indiciated that epidemiology mainly deals with data derived from nonexperimental studies. Nonetheless, it is instructive to consider in some detail several experimental studies on human populations.

1. The University Group Diabetes Program (UGDP)

Diabetes is a disease of varying severity for which various treatment methods are available. For mild disease, control of dietary sugar intake may be all that is prescribed. For moderate disease, treatment with oral agents that lower blood sugar is usual. For severe disease, treatment with insulin is usual. However, there is a wide spectrum of moderate disease, and individual physicians may treat individual patients with any of the three general methods.

The primary goal of treating diabetics is to keep the blood sugar level within the normal range. The ultimate goal is to prevent early death from the sequellae of diabetes, mainly cardiovascular disease. While it is supposed that lowering blood sugar leads to a reduced mortality in general and to reduced mortality from cardiovascular disease specifically, this has not been demonstrated conclusively.

In 1960, a study was designed with three objectives:[7]

1. Evaluation of the efficacy of hypoglycemic treatments in the prevention of vascular complications in a long-term, prospective, and cooperative clinical trial
2. Study of the natural history of vascular disease in maturity onset, noninsulin dependent diabetics
3. Development of methods applicable to cooperative clinical trials

An experiment (clinical trial) was ethical because each of the three methods of treatment was in current use and none was clearly superior. (This is the usual situation, also, whenever a new treatment is developed that has promise of being better than existing treatments.) Thus there was no general opposition to the setting-up of this trial.

Twelve diabetes clinics in twelve cities took part in the study. Patients with diabetes diagnosed within the previous year, who did not require insulin therapy to remain symptom-free, and who had a reasonable likelihood of living at least five years were eligible for entrance into the study. All eligible patients were told the nature of the study and were asked if they would be willing to participate. Only those who were willing to be treated with any one of the three possible modes of treatment were enrolled.

One of five types of therapy was assigned at random to each patient: diet only, diet plus one of two types of oral hypoglycemic agent, or diet plus one of two types of insulin therapy. By assigning treatment at random, all factors that were related to the risk of death from cardiovascular disease, except for the treatment, tended to be distributed equally across the three groups. This random assignment of exposure (treatment) was the primary means of controlling potential *confounding bias*. However, there was no guarantee that one group might, by chance, have a higher baseline risk of death than the others. Factors related to the probability of dying such as age, sex, blood cholesterol level, degree of current cardiovascular disease, cigarette smoking habit, etc. were not necessarily randomly distributed. However, in general, gross disparities should not result from the process of randomization.

Absolute control of potential *observation bias* was not possible between the insulin-treated patients and the others. Since insulin can be given only by syringe, blind treatment was not possible. However, *blindness* was possible between the diet and the oral hypoglycemic groups. Persons on diet only were given placebo pills identical in appearance to the oral hypoglycemic pills. Since neither the patient nor the physician knew which pill was the placebo and which was the hypoglycemic, the study was *double-blind*. In the assessment of cause of death, i.e., cardiovascular disease or not, the knowledge of exposure could not bias the physician's decision as to the cause of death.

Objectivity was also used in assessing death. Outcome was measured not only as to cause of death but as to fact of death. While there may be disagreement as to the pathologic process that led to death, there is no question as to whether a person has died. Therefore, total mortality as well as cause-specific mortality comparisions were made between the insulin-treated groups and those treated with oral therapy only.

No *selection bias* was possible because the disease (death) had not occurred when the assignment of exposure was made.

Patients were enrolled into the study between 1961 and 1966. By October, 1969, the mortality data in Table 3.5 had been collected. (Data from only one of the two insulin-treated groups are presented). The death rates from cardiovascular disease and from all causes are seen to be higher in the group treated with oral hypoglycemic agents than in the other two groups.

The data resulting from this experimental study gave rise to a controversy that remains today. The belief at the time the study was set up was that, if anything, oral hypoglycemic agents and insulin both would lead to a reduced mortality in relation to the diet only group. The excess mortality among the oral agent group was quite unexpected. As a result, these data have been thoroughly examined and reanalyzed and a number of criticisms have been made.[8,9]

Among the criticisms are questions about the baseline comparability of the five treatment groups. Even though assignment of treatment was random, there were differences in the percentage of "cardiovascular risk factors" among groups. Specifically, persons assigned to the oral hypoglycemic agent treatment group had more persons with high cholesterol levels, with obesity, who were male, etc. Further, data on an important risk factor — cigarette smoking — were not even collected.

Thus, even though this was an experiment where randomization was possible, questions were raised about the adequacy of the control of potential confounding bias. A number of reanalyses of the data have been carried out, and the original authors still belive that the data strongly suggest an adverse outcome in the treatment of diabetics with oral hypoglycemic agents. This belief, however, is disputed by many physicians in clinical practice.

There is little controversy as to whether the results were flawed because of observation bias. The decision as to whether a person died from cardiovascular causes was made without knowledge of the person's treatment. The decision as to whether a person died was unambiguous.

2. Hospitalization after Myocardial Infarction

At one time persons who had a heart attack and survived were kept in the hospital for up to 6 weeks. As time went by, this period was reduced to 3 weeks. The determi-

Table 3.5
DEATHS FROM CARDIOVASCULAR CAUSES AND FROM ALL CAUSES AMONG DIABETICS TREATED BY THREE METHODS

A. Cardiovascular causes

Treatment group	Deceased			Rate
	Yes	No	Total	
Diet only	10	195	205	4.9/100
Oral agent	26	178	204	12.7/100
Insulin	13	197	210	6.2/100

B. All causes

Treatment group	Deceased			Rate
	Yes	No	Total	
Diet only	21	184	205	10.2/100
Oral agent	30	174	204	14.7/100
Insulin	20	190	210	9.5/100

nation of how long a period of hospitalization was necessary following a heart attack was dictated largely by the common practice of clinicians.

In the early 1970s, an experiment was designed to evaluate whether a 3-week stay in the hospital was any better (or worse) than a 2-week stay.[10] The motivation was largely practical; the cost of hospitalization was and is increasing at a rapid rate.

Persons with an uncomplicated myocardial infarction and whose physician agreed to the study were assigned either a 2-week or a 3-week in-hospital recovery period. To control potential confounding, both matching and randomization were done. First, patients were divided into six age-sex groups. Next, an envelope was selected assigning the patient to either the 2-week or the 3-week hospital stay period. The assignment was random in that, for each pair of patients of the same age and sex, each had an equal probability of being assigned to the 2-week or the 3-week group.

After a 24 week follow-up period, the results were as presented in Table 3.6. Clearly, there was no evidence that persons hospitalized only 2 weeks had a poorer outcome.

Again, even though this was an experiment, questions may be raised about confounding bias and observation bias. No confounding from age and sex was possible, since they were matched in the study design. By definition, therefore, they were not associated with exposure (2- or 3-week treatment). There were differences, however. Of the 2-week patients 17% had had a previous heart attack in comparison to only 12% of the 3-week patients. However, since a previous heart attack would seem to be a positive risk factor for a subsequent bad outcome (e.g., death), this difference could not account for the results seen in Table 3.6. If anything, the 2-week patients had a better outcome than the 3-week patients.

Observation bias, however, was quite possible. The patients could not be blinded as to the length of their hospital stay. Returning to work is clearly a subjective measure of improvement. Arguments can be made that either the 2-week or the 3-week patients would be more likely to return to work early because of their knowledge of the length of hospital stay. Death, of course, is not subject to this bias.

Table 3.6
OUTCOME AT 24 WEEKS AFTER
AN UNCOMPLICATED HEART
ATTACK

Outcome

Returned to work

Treatment	Yes	No	Total	Rate
Two-week	40	29	69	58/100
Three-week	34	35	69	49/100

Developed new symptoms

Two-week	6	63	69	9/100
Three-week	6	63	69	9/100

Died

Two-week	3	66	69	4/100
Three-week	5	64	69	7/100

3. Comment

Data resulting from an experiment are usually considered superior to data resulting from a nonexperiment. This is because of the ability of an investigator to assign exposure at random and therefore to minimize confounding bias. That this is no guarantee, however, is clear from the controversy surrounding the UGDP. Also, the possibility that observation bias can affect the measure of the occurrence of disease is present in all types of studies.

The design of an experimental study is a model for a nonexperimental epidemiologic study. However, there is no clear-cut parallel between experimental:good and nonexperimental:bad. All types of studies on human (or animal) populations are subject to error and to bias. Many methods used to prevent or control such problems are used both in experimental and in nonexperimental studies.

B. Descriptive Studies

In the definition of a descriptive study, information on both cause and effect in an individual is *not* available. Descriptive studies are mainly confined to the presentation of routinely collected data. These data may be health-related, for example, vital statistics on birth or death, or collected for other reasons, for example, cigarette sales per capita.

Descriptive data by themselves usually can not be used as the basis for a change in behavior related to health or as the critical evidence in deciding that a substance causes a disease. Because data on individuals are not available, the relationship between exposure and disease is indirect.

1. Cigarette Smoking and Lung Cancer

By 1945 it was apparent from Vital Statistics data that the mortality rate from lung cancer among males was increasing (Figure 3.3).[11] The percentage of cigarette smokers was also increasing with time (Figure 3.4).[12] The meaning of these descriptive studies is not clear. Many other factors can be shown to have increased over the same period (percent of homes with refrigerators, percent of population living in an urban area,

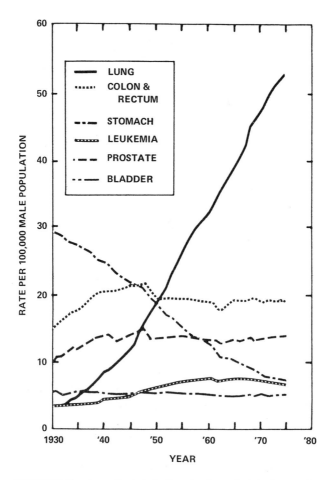

FIGURE 3.3. Age-adjusted death rates for selected sites, males,
U.S., 1930-1975.

percent of persons with automobiles). To say that these data show that cigarette smoking is a cause of lung cancer would be an over-interpretation.

The descriptive data in Figure 3.5 are somewhat more convincing.[13] However, cigarettes sold per capita probably are related to other factors (annual income, alcohol consumption, religious preference). A number of potential confounding factors can be postulated.

2. County of Residence and Mortality from Cancer

In 1974, the National Cancer Institute published an atlas of mortality rates of specific cancers for each county in the United States.[14] As an exercise in descriptive epidemiology, this atlas is of great value. The data can be used to compare cancer mortality in one area to that in another. Counties with certain characteristics can be selected and examined. For example, counties where the chemical industry is highly concentrated have excess mortality rates of bladder, lung, and liver cancers.[15] This association can be examined further to assess the possibility that working in or living nearby a chemical plant is responsible for the excess cancer. However, on the basis of these descriptive data, no definitive relationship between the chemical industry and cancer can be established.

These data have been used to examine the relationship between drinking water and

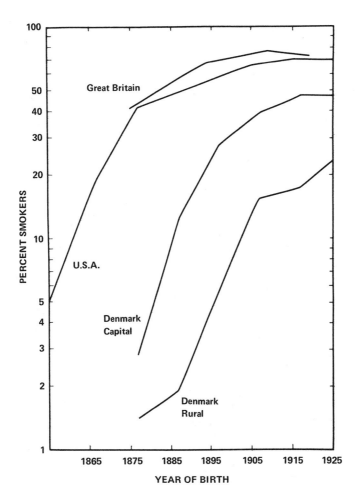

FIGURE 3.4.   Percent smokers according to year of birth in three countries.

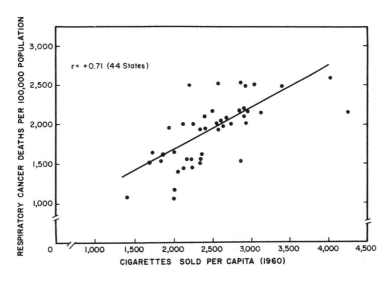

FIGURE 3.5.   Association between respiratory cancer mortality for U.S. residents and annual cigarette sales.

cancer. The cancer rates in the New Orleans area are in excess. A number of chemicals that are carcinogenic in animals have been found in the drinking water of New Orleans. The suggestion has been made that the chemicals in the water, which are present in very low concentrations, are responsible for the excess cancer mortality.[16]

Whether chemicals in the New Orleans drinking water cause cancer in the persons who drink the water is unknown. However, to conclude that the descriptive epidemiologic data indicate a health hazard from drinking water is not possible. At a minimum, it is necessary to evaluate the possible effects of confounding factors.

3. Comment

Descriptive data on human populations are an important part of epidemiology. Many patterns have been seen in such data that have aided in the understanding of the cause of disease (e.g., Farr's data on cholera). To ignore such data is to ignore the basic characteristics of human populations.

However, such data are at the opposite pole from data collected in the experimental setting. The epidemiologist has no control over how the data are collected and has no knowledge of the factors leading to bias in the data. To use descriptive data as the sole basis for decisions on human health is not possible.

Consider the potential for bias in county-specific death rates. These data have their source in the death certificate made out at the time of death. Some examples of the possible errors include:

1. Smokers with respiratory disease may be said to have died from lung cancer; nonsmokers with respiratory disease may be said to have died from pneumonia.
2. Counties with chemical industries may have a high foreign-born population; foreign-born persons may have a high rate of liver cancer.
3. Physicians in New Orleans may detect or diagnose cancer at an earlier stage than physicians in the rest of the country; data from the autopsy may appear on the death certificate in New Orleans more frequently than on death certificates in the rest of the country.

The possibility for observation bias and/or confounding bias to be present in data resulting from a descriptive study is at least as great as the possibility in an experiment. Moreover, it is more difficult in a descriptive study than in an experiment to understand or even detect such bias. It is essential that descriptive data neither be discarded nor embraced without reservation. Such data are part of the spectrum of information on health in human populations.

C. Prospective Cohort Studies

Prospective cohort studies are similar in appearance to experimental studies (see Figure 3.2). The investigator is present at the time exposed and nonexposed groups are defined; the investigator then ages along with the study population. Because of the necessity for time to pass in order for disease to develop, experimental and prospective cohort studies frequently require many years for completion.

However, there is a major difference between experimental and prospective cohort studies. In an experiment, the investigator has complete control over which persons are assigned to "exposed" and "not exposed" groups. Because of this control, exposure can be essentially random; factors that may be associated with the risk of disease tend to be equally distributed between the exposed and not exposed group and therefore tend not to be confounding.

In prospective cohort studies, no control over exposure is possible. Persons are selected to be included in the study on the basis of past or current exposure or nonexposure. The investigator has no role in deciding whether an individual is exposed. Consequently, it is possible that other causes of the disease(s) under study are associated with the exposure and thus are confounding. If an association is found between an exposure and a disease, it may reflect a direct causal association or an indirect association due to confounding. (This is also true in an experiment, but the likelihood is lower). Consequently, in prospective cohort studies efforts must be made to identify all factors associated with exposure.

Another difference between prospective cohort and experimental studies lies in the degree to which blindness is possible. In an experimental study of a drug, it is possible to treat one group with a drug and the other group with an identical placebo. Neither the patient nor his physician know which treatment is being received, and consequently no observation bias is possible in the definition of outcome.

In prospective cohort studies, this absolute blindness is not possible. The persons in the study may not know the reason for the study, and the physician measuring the outcome may not know to which study group an individual belongs. However, someone at some time knows something about an individual's exposure status; consequently, absolute blindness cannot be guaranteed.

Objectivity in the measure of disease occurrence can be made the same in a prospective cohort study as in an experiment. The person diagnosing outcome can use identical criteria in exposed and nonexposed groups.

1. The Honolulu Heart Study

During the period 1965—68, 7705 men of Japanese ancestry without diagnosed heart disease were entered into a prospective cohort study in Hawaii.[17] On entrance into the study, information was collected on characteristics thought to be related to the subsequent development of heart disease. Also, information was collected on a person's diet, including coffee and alcohol intake.

An attempt was made to follow all 7705 men at least 6 years. Reexaminations were scheduled on the second and the sixth anniversary of enrollment. New cases of heart disease were ascertained by these reexaminations as well as by search of hospital and vital statistics records.

At the conclusion of 6 years of follow-up, incidence rates of heart disease were computed for groups with differing base-line characteristics of coffee and of alcohol consumption. As seen in Table 3.7, men who drank three or more cups of coffee per day had higher rates of heart disease than men who drank two or fewer cups. As seen in Table 3.8, the more alcohol consumed per day, the lower the rate of heart disease.

There was a positive association between cigarette smoking and coffee consumption and between cigarette smoking and heart disease. After control for cigarette smoking, no association between coffee intake and heart disease was seen. In contrast, no confounding factors could be identified to explain the negative association between alcohol consumption and coronary artery disease. The occurrence of heart disease was ascertained without knowledge of a person's coffee or alcohol habits.

A major problem in the conduct of prospective cohort studies such as this is that persons initially enrolled tend to leave the study or become "lost-to-follow-up". In order to compute incidence rates of disease at the completion of the study, the length of time each person was being followed must be known. Ideally, in this study each man would have been followed 6 years or until the occurrence of heart disease, whichever came first. However, some persons move, some become disenchanted with the study, and some are too busy to be reexamined. If investigators are unable to maintain contact with each individual the person-years of follow-up become imprecise. Since

Table 3.7

SIX-YEAR INCIDENCE RATE OF
HEART DISEASE ACCORDING TO
COFFEE INTAKE

Coffee intake[a]	Men at risk	Incidence rate[b]
0	1235	32.4
1—2	2484	31.7
3—4	2068	43.3
5 +	1918	43.5

[a] Cups/day.
[b] Cases/1000/6 years. Age-adjusted.

these person-years are needed to compute the incidence rate of heart disease, the measure of disease occurrence is also imprecise.

If the percentage of persons lost-to-follow-up does not differ materially between persons with different alcohol consumption habits, it may be expected that the incidence rates of heart disease in the alcohol-consumption groups are affected to roughly the same extent by any losses. Whereas the rates computed may differ from the actual rates of occurrence, any error will affect each alcohol-specific rate to roughly the same extent. However, if there is a greater percentage of loss for heavy alcohol consumers than for light consumers, the data seen in Table 3.8 might result. If it is assumed that all persons could have been followed for the full 6 years (except for those who develop disease), and if progressively heavier alcohol users had a progressively greater loss-to-follow-up, then there would have been progressive under-ascertainment of heart disease in the heavier users.

In the study cited, there is no reason to believe that such losses, in fact, accounted for the negative association between alcohol consumption and heart attack. Further, if there were losses, each person should not be considered to contribute a full 6 person-years. Rather, he would be considered to be under follow-up only for as long as he was, in fact, known to be free from heart disease. Thus, even though there were differential loss according to alcohol consumption, the difference could be adjusted for by comparing the number of cases of heart disease by the actual person-years followed rather than by the potential person-years followed.

2. The Collaborative Perinatal Project (CPP)

During the period 1959—65, 55,908 pregnant women were entered into a prospective cohort study in 12 medical centers in the United States. On entrance into the study, information was collected on basic characteristics relating to pregnancy, including medications being used. Each woman was followed until the pregnancy was completed. At specified periods following entrance, information was obtained about other characteristics related to the pregnancy, including birth defects occurring in the child.

A number of studies have been done or are in progress on the data obtained from the CPP. In one, an analysis was made of the relation between drugs taken during pregnancy and birth defects in the offspring.[18] Of the women entered into the study, 50,282 were included in this analysis.

Of the 55,908 women registered, over 2,000 refused to participate. Since these women technically were never in the study, there is little concern that their refusal led to any important bias. Another 954 pregnancies resulted in termination before the 20th week of pregnancy; no information was thus available on birth defects in fetuses who did not reach a viable age (20 weeks). Finally, 1695 pregnancies were excluded because

Table 3.8
SIX-YEAR INCIDENCE RATE OF
HEART DISEASE ACCORDING TO
ALCOHOL INTAKE

Alcohol intake[a]	Men at risk	Incidence rate[b]
0	3565	46.0
1—6	1034	41.2
7—15	962	30.7
16—39	1024	26.7
40 +	1006	21.2

[a] ml/day.
[b] Cases/1000/6 years. Age-adjusted.

of special characteristics (multiple births, ethnic group other than white, black, or Puerto Rican), or because of missing baseline data. The remaining 50,282 women were followed at least to the completion of their pregnancy.

Losses-to-follow-up were much less of a concern in this study than in the Honolulu Heart Study. The period of potential follow-up was no more than 9 months; the outcome of interest of necessity had to occur in a limited time period; the reasons for exclusion were mainly based on information available at the time the women were entered into the study.

The length of time needed to conduct this study was determined not by the years needed for a disease to develop, but by the years needed to enroll the projected number of women. In theory, at least, the enrollment period could have been made much shorter simply by expanding the number of medical centers that were participating. Thus a prospective cohort study of pregnancy does not necessarily require many years to complete.

No specific hypotheses were set up prior to the study. The general aims were many; one was to evaluate the relationship between drugs in pregnancy and birth defects. This was a large task. There were several hundred different drugs used and several hundred different birth defects that occurred. Of importance was the potential for confounding. Each drug was given for a specific purpose — the treatment of some symptom or disease. Thus, if an association between a drug and a birth defect were found, it would be difficult to separate the association between the drug and the defect from the association between the disease and the defect. This high degree of potential confounding was not apparent in the Honolulu Heart Study.

Also, it is difficult in this situation to assess the potential for observation bias. Women in the study were under the usual care of an obstetrician. The obstetrician was responsible for the prenatal care of the woman and for the prescribing of any medication. The obstetrician, along with a pediatrician, made the diagnosis of any birth defect in the child. Since many defects are relatively minor and subject to differences of opinion, it is possible that some defect may have been over-diagnosed in women with certain treated medical conditions of pregnancy. Such observation bias would be beyond the control (or knowledge) of the investigator.

The data in Tables 2.2 and 2.3 are from the CPP. Phenytoin is a drug used to control epilepsy. An association between phenytoin and congenital malformations was identified. However, since most women who received phenytoin also were epileptic, it is possible that congenital malformations occurred in children born to epileptic women rather than to those who received phenytoin. Clearly, an experimental study would be much more powerful than a prospective cohort study in evaluating the independent associations of phenytoin and of epilepsy with congenital malformations.

Observation bias, also, is a concern in the evaluation of the association between phenytoin and birth defects. Once a suspicion has been raised that phenytoin causes birth defects, children born to epileptic women taking phenytoin are subject to greater scrutiny for birth defects. Relatively minor defects may be diagnosed (or over-diagnosed) in children born to women taking phenytoin and under-diagnosed in children born to other women.

Note that in the data in Table 2.3, incidence rates were not used as the measure of disease frequency. Rather, prevalence rates were computed (cases/100 children). The denominator is children, not children-years.

3. Comment

Prospective cohort studies usually require much time and money. Consequently, such studies are usually not the initial step in the evaluation of a specific question. Rather, prospective cohort studies are used to explore general factors related to disease such as what are the determinants of heart disease or what characteristics of pregnancy are related to what abnormal outcome of pregnancy. Also, groups of persons with specific exposures can be studied. A number of prospective cohort studies have been done of cigarette smokers.[19-21]

Few prospective cohort studies have been done in occupational settings. Many are being planned or are in progress. Until recently, most concerns about adverse effects on health of working in industry have been with acute illness following shortly after exposure to a specific substance. Such associations can be readily recognized in the clinical setting. However, with the current concern as to the possible occurrence of cancer and other chronic diseases many years after employment in industry, much effort is being devoted to developing data on employees that may be used in the future. The recording of data on work exposures and on personal habits and characteristics is the beginning of a prospective cohort study.

D. Retrospective Cohort Studies

In contrast to prospective cohort studies, retrospective cohort studies have been extensively carried out in occupational settings. A variety of records are maintained by industries that contain information on a person's work history. Since it usually is possible to estimate which substances have been used in which work areas, it is possible to define a cohort of workers on the basis of exposure in the past. Using records maintained by the company as well as other records such as death certificates, the cohort can be followed to the present to ascertain the occurrence of disease. Most frequently, only diseases appearing on the death certificate can be identified.

There are several major differences between a prospective cohort study and a retrospective cohort study:

1. Since the study population is being followed from some time in the past to the present, the length of time needed for the study tends to be shorter in a retrospective cohort study.
2. Much less detail on a person's characteristics or exposures are available in a retrospective cohort study. In a prospective cohort study in industry, the investigator can collect data on smoking, drinking, eating, current diseases, etc. as well as a detailed picture of industrial exposures; in a retrospective cohort study, all that is usually available is a rough idea as to a person's work history.
3. In a prospective cohort study, the investigator usually compares disease rates between two or more groups (smoker vs. nonsmoker, heavy drinker vs. moderate drinker vs. nondrinker). In a retrospective cohort study, there frequently is no formal comparison group. Rather, mortality rates among the exposed group are compared to the mortality rates of some general population.

4.   In prospective cohort studies, exposures of today are being evaluated; in retro-
      spective cohort studies the exposures of perhaps 30 to 50 years ago are being
      evaluated.

While there is no question that a prospective cohort study provides more reliable
data, the short-comings of retrospective cohort studies do not render them useless. A
person's work exposures tend to be relatively nonassociated with other determinants
of disease; consequently, the potential for confounding by unmeasured factors is not
overwhelming. Mortality rates on general populations have been shown emperically to
be useful bases of comparison. Exposures of today frequently are similar to those of
yesterday.

In general, however, confounding bias is less amenable to control in retrospective
cohort studies than in prospective cohort studies. Therefore, interpretation of data
from retrospective cohort studies must always be cautious. Usually, it is not possible
to obtain data on factors (e.g., smoking) that are likely to be associated with the risk
of disease.

Observation bias, also, is more difficult to prevent in a retrospective cohort study.
If a mortality study is being conducted, the definition of disease is done by a person
other than the investigator. Usually, no information is available as to the process that
led to the diagnosis of the cause of death. Conceivably, certain symptoms in one group
are diagnosed differently from the same symptoms in a second group.

Perhaps the best way to evaluate whether an association seen in a retrospective cohort study is due to bias is to replicate the study in another group with a similar exposure. Preferably, the replication should be done by another investigator. If similar
associations are seen in different studies of different groups done by different investigators with different biases, then the belief that the associations are causal is strengthened.

1. Mortality Among Steelworkers

In 1962, a mortality study among 59,072 steelworkers was begun. These were all the
men employed in 1953 at seven iron and steel producing plants in Allegheny County,
Pennsylvania.[22] Between July 1962 and December 1964, clerks visited each of these
plants and abstracted basic data on each of the workers. The data included social
security number, race, date of birth, employment information (job title and dates employed in each job), all addresses at which the worker lived, and information on next
of kin. Over the next several years an attempt was made to determine the vital status
of each individual as of 12/31/1961; each person was identified on that date as being
alive, deceased or lost-to-follow-up.

The follow-up of persons in a retrospective cohort study requires much effort. A
variety of sources must be used.[23] In this study, a search was made of current employee
records, county death lists, R. L. Polk and telephone directories, post office sources,
the Internal Revenue Service, the Social Security Administration, telephone contacts,
the Board of Public Assistance, the Bureau of Employment Security, and the Bureau
of Missing Persons. Of the 59,072 steelworkers in this study, 4716 were found to have
died, 54,259 were found to be alive and only 97 (0.2%) were lost-to-follow-up. This
high follow-up was desired so that no assumption need be made in computing mortality
rates among the steelworkers.

Mortality rates from several causes of death are presented in Table 3.9 for white
and nonwhite steelworkers compared to white and nonwhite residents of Allegheny
County. For each ethnic group, the mortality rates in the steelworkers are considerably
lower than the rates for members of the general population.

Table 3.9

MORTALITY RATES FOR WHITE AND NONWHITE STEELWORKERS IN COMPARISON TO MORTALITY RATES FOR WHITE AND BLACK RESIDENTS OF ALLEGHENY COUNTY, PA.

Ethnic group	Cause of death	Mortality rates[a]	
		Steelworkers	Allegheny County
White	All	9.1	15.8
	Heart disease	3.4	6.1
	Respiratory disease	0.3	0.6
Nonwhite	All	9.9	18.8
	Heart disease	2.2	4.9
	Respiratory disease	0.5	1.1

[a]   Deaths/1000/year.

The data in Table 3.9 are "crude" rates. That is, the numbers of deaths among steelworkers were simply divided by the number of person-years of follow-up to obtain the crude mortality rates (incidence-type rates). Also, the data for Allegheny County residents were crude rates. However, if there were a difference in the age-distributions of the steelworkers and of the County residents, age would be confounding, since age clearly is related to the mortality rate. One way to control for such confounding is to compute the number of deaths expected among steelworkers on the basis of the age-specific rates of the Allegheny County residents. The results of such computations are presented in Table 3.10.

It can be seen that while there was some confounding by age, the numbers of deaths among the steelworkers are still less than those expected on the basis of general population rates. The presence of confounding by age can be inferred, since in Table 3.9 the ratio of steelworker to county rates of all causes of death is 0.58 for whites and 0.53 for nonwhites. In Table 3.10, the ratio of observed to expected deaths is 0.86 for whites and 0.64 for nonwhites.

This overall lower death rate in steelworkers relative to the general population is a frequent finding and has been termed the "healthy worker effect". This is somewhat of a misnomer, since similar deficits are found when other nonhospitalized groups are followed, e.g., religious groups. A more general term would be "healthy person effect". General populations are made up of two groups: the healthy and the ill. Those who are healthy tend to be employed and those who are ill tend to be hospitalized. Each, however, contributes to the overall mortality rate of the general population.

The healthy worker effect is an example of confounding bias. Persons of good general health status are selected to be employed in industry. Because good health status is associated with outcome (a lower risk of dying) and with exposure (employment in industry), it meets the definition of confounding.

The healthy worker effect is not an example of selection bias, even though healthy persons are "selected" for employment. Selection bias in the steelworkers study, or any in retrospective cohort study, would occur if persons with disease were selectively entered into the study cohort. For example, if an evaluation is being made of the association between beryllium and lung cancer, selection bias would result if persons with lung cancer who had worked with beryllium would be selectively enrolled into the study group in preference to persons without lung cancer who had worked with beryllium.

Table 3.10
NUMBERS OF DEATHS OBSERVED BETWEEN
1953 AND 1961 AMONG WHITE AND NONWHITE
STEELWORKERS AND NUMBERS EXPECTED
BASED ON AGE-ETHNIC GROUP — SPECIFIC
MORTALITY RATES OF ALLEGHENY COUNTY
MALES

Ethnic group	Cause of death	Numbers of deaths	
		Observed	Expected
White	All	4083	4773.5
	Heart disease	1537	1773.4
	Respiratory disease	136	178.4
Nonwhite	All	633	993.3
	Heart disease	143	229.5
	Respiratory disease	29	59.2

One feature of retrospective cohort studies is that they tend to become "prospective" as time goes by. This is also somewhat of a misnomer, since the basic information at cohort definition is all that is used for definition of exposure. However, after an initial analysis, the investigator may age along with the cohort and wait for further diseases to develop or deaths to occur. This was the case in the steelworkers study.[24]

As seen in Table 3.11, among coke plant workers, excess lung cancer was seen in those who worked on the coke ovens while no excess lung cancer was seen among nonoven workers. In these data the expected numbers were computed on the basis of lung cancer rates among all steelworkers rather than on the basis of rates among the general population. In so doing, the confounding bias of the healthy worker effect was controlled. The lung cancer rates in the "healthy" steelworkers were used as a basis of comparison for the coke plant workers. Unless some source of bias can be detected with respect to coke oven workers, these data seem to show that working in the coke oven section of the coke plant is a cause of lung cancer.

Further elaboration of these data is presented in Chapter 9.

2. Breast Cancer Following Fluoroscopic Examination of the Chest

In the 1930s and 1940s, tuberculosis of the lung was a common disease with no effective treatment. One means of treatment was air-collapse therapy: air was injected between the lung and the chest wall so as to collapse the lung. It was believed that by resting the lung, healing would proceed faster. Because the air gradually was absorbed, frequent refills were needed. During each refill, the degree of lung collapse was monitored by a fluoroscope. In so doing, considerable radiation was given to the chest area.

Currently, there is interest in the early detection of breast cancer by means of X-ray mammography. It is hoped that early detection with concomitant early treatment will result in lower mortality rates from breast cancer. However, there is concern that the radiation received in mammography may itself cause breast cancer.

To evaluate the association between radiation to the breast and the subsequent development of breast cancer, a retrospective cohort study was done.[4] Women aged 13 to 40 who were treated for tuberculosis in selected Massachusetts sanatoria between 1930 and 1954 were identified. The study cohort consisted of 1047 women who had been treated with air-collapse therapy and 717 women who received other treatments.

Extensive follow-up of these women was carried out.[25] Of the 1764 women in the

Table 3.11
NUMBERS OF DEATHS OBSERVED BETWEEN 1953 AND 1966 AMONG COKE PLANT WORKERS AND NUMBERS EXPECTED BASED ON AGE-SPECIFIC MORTALITY RATES OF THE STEELWORKERS

| | Location within coke plant | | | |
| | Coke oven | | Nonoven | |
Cause of death	Observed	Expected	Observed	Expected
All causes	214	192.4	178	163.5
All cancers	75	43.9	43	34.6
Lung cancer	40	14.1	5	9.7

study, 505 were found to have died, 1146 were found to be alive and 113 (6.4%) were lost-to-follow-up. The percentage lost was similar in the exposed group (5.2%) and in the nonexposed group (8.2%). While the follow-up was made without knowledge of exposure status, so as to minimize observation bias, it is reassuring that the percentages lost did not differ greatly.

The occurrence of breast cancer is presented in Table 3.12. As in the steelworkers study, two methods of comparison were used:

1. An external comparison was made with incidence rates of the Connecticut Tumor Registry; among the women treated with air collapse therapy, an excess of breast cancer was seen while among the comparison women there was no excess.
2. The crude incidence rate of breast cancer in the exposed women was twice the rate in the nonexposed women. In each method an excess of breast cancer was seen among the women treated with air collapse therapy.

As part of the data collection process, a questionnaire was sent to women who were found to be alive. Information was obtained on breast cancer history and on a number of factors associated with tuberculosis or with the risk of developing breast cancer. Data on several of these characteristics are presented in Table 3.13. Isoniazid therapy was more common among the women treated with air collapse therapy. However, since Isoniazid was shown not to be associated with breast cancer, it could not be confounding. Family history of breast cancer, benign breast disease, and having no children are factors that frequently are more common in women with breast disease. However, since each of these factors shows little association with exposure, little or no confounding is possible.

Observation bias seems unlikely in this study. The ascertainment of breast cancer was obtained either from death certificates or from a mail questionnaire. The physician who filled out the death certificate probably was unaware that the women had been treated with air collapse therapy many years previously. The woman herself was not told the specific reason for the study in the letter accompanying the questionnaire. While the impetus for the study came from the interest in the association between radiation exposure received during air collapse therapy and breast cancer, the study itself was a general evaluation of morbidity and mortality following treatment for tuberculosis.

3. Comment

The occupational setting lends itself naturally to the retrospective cohort study. In

Table 3.12
OCCURRENCE OF BREAST CANCER IN
WOMEN WITH TUBERCULOSIS
ACCORDING TO MODE OF TREATMENT

Treatment	Number of women	Breast cancer		
		Observed	Expected[a]	Rate[b]
Air collapse therapy	1047	41	23.3	1.5
Other	717	15	14.1	0.8

[a] Expected numbers computed on basis of age-year specific incidence rates for Connecticut women.
[b] Number of breast cancers/1000 women/year.

Table 3.13
PERCENTAGE OF SELECTED
CHARACTERISTICS IN WOMEN TREATED
WITH AIR COLLAPSE THERAPY AND IN
COMPARISON WOMEN

Characteristic	Treatment	
	Air collapse therapy	Other
Isoniazid therapy	29.0	17.4
Family history of breast cancer	6.1	6.3
Benign breast disease	15.5	13.9
Nulliparous	28.4	24.1

order to evaluate the relationship between work and disease (or health), an important source of information is the personnel records from the past. One task of the occupational epidemiologist is to search for such old records. Equally important is the preservation of records. Frequently, in the spirit of economy or of modernization, old industrial or medical records are scheduled for destruction. Yet, as illustrated in these two studies, these records have value beyond their original use.

Lessons learned from retrospective cohort studies should be used in designing prospective cohort studies. The records of today must be preserved for tomorrow. Information of potential use to the epidemiologist of tomorrow must be entered onto the records of today. Provisions must be made today to find people tomorrow.

E. Case-Control Studies

Case-control studies are frequently termed "retrospective" studies because one is looking backward from disease to exposure. This contrast with cohort studies which have been called "prospective" because one looks forward from exposure to disease. However, simply referring to a study as retrospective or prospective leads to confusion, especially in discussing retrospective cohort studies. Here, one is looking forward from exposure to disease, but the study utilizes past data. Further, in many case-control studies, data to be collected in the future are used. Since retrospective and prospective are ambiguous terms, they should be used only to modify a more basic type of study.

In a case-control study, the investigation selects persons with the disease of interest as the "cases" and other persons as the "controls". Not infrequently, more than one disease is of interest, so there may be a number of case groups. Also, the controls may either be persons with other diseases or persons with no known disease. In the simplest situation, however, the cases are persons with a specific disease and the controls are persons without that disease.

In general, case-control studies evaluate a number of exposures in relation to one disease. Cohort studies evaluate a number of diseases in relation to one exposure. A rule of thumb is that if the disease is rare, a case-control study is more efficient to do because persons with the disease can be sought out and selectively enrolled. Likewise, if the exposure is rare a cohort study is more efficient because exposed persons can be selectively identified. Case-control studies tend to be done in hospital populations because that is where persons with disease congregate.

Two general types of control groups are used in case-control studies: hospital controls and population controls. As emphasized earlier, epidemiologists are always concerned with comparability. Hospital controls and cases are similar in that each group is comprised of persons in the hospital. The reasons for hospitalization, the data on diagnostic procedures, and the milieu of the data gathering tend to be comparable. However, there may be concern that one disease group is selectively admitted to a hospital. For example, all persons with an acute heart attack tend to be hospitalized, while only a small percentage of persons with arthritis enter the hospital. In a study of arthritis, population controls may be preferable in that their demographic characteristics and day-to-day habits may be more comparable to the cases. Neither type of control group is necessarily preferable in a given case-control study.

1. Bladder Cancer in the Greater Boston Area

Between 1/1/67 and 6/30/68, an effort was made to identify all newly diagnosed persons with bladder cancer in the Greater Boston area.[26] Through a review of the pathology logs in 111 hospitals, 668 persons were identified with bladder cancer. Because this was a population-based study, it was possible to compute the annual incidence rate of bladder cancer.

Controls were selected from Massachusetts Residents Lists that are updated annually. First, several thousand names were drawn at random from the Residents Lists such that the proportion from a given city was the same as the proportion from that city in the general population. Then, for each case, a control of the same sex and same year of birth was selected.

For reasons of economy, interviews were attempted with about only 500 each of the cases and controls. Successful interviews at home were completed with 96.3% of the cases and 93.6% of the controls. Questions included information on smoking, coffee drinking, and occupation.

As seen in Table 3.14, in both men and women a greater percent of cases than of controls reported having been a regular cigarette smoker. Note that the percentage of smokers among cases and controls is presented rather than the rate of bladder cancer in smokers and nonsmokers. The rate of bladder cancer (50%) in this table has no meaning since the ratio of cases to controls was set arbitrarily at 1:1. However, the percentage of smokers within each group is not affected by the ratio of cases to controls.

Because the age and sex distributions of the cases and controls were made to be similar in the design of the study, no confounding by these factors is possible. They are not related to the disease in the study data even though they are undoubtedly related to cigarette smoking. However, there may be other cases of bladder cancer more common among smokers than among nonsmokers that could account for the association with bladder cancer.

Table 3.14
RELATIONSHIP BETWEEN BLADDER CANCER
AND REGULAR CIGARETTE SMOKING IN
GREATER BOSTON[a]

	Men				Women		
		Bladder cancer				Bladder cancer	
Cigarette smoker	Yes	No		Cigarette smoker	Yes	No	
Yes	286	247		Yes	55	37	
No	70	109		No	50	68	
Total	356	356		Total	105	105	
Percentage smoker	80	69		Percentage smoker	52	35	

[a] Data modified from Reference 26.

Observation bias is quite possible, in that both the interviewers and patients knew who was a case and who was a control. It is possible that cases over-reported smoking cigarettes or that controls under-reported the habit. In order to minimize this possibility, the questions asked of the cases and controls were objective and close-ended. No suggestion was made that the study was being done to show that smoking caused bladder cancer. Rather, the study was presented as, and indeed was, an evaluation of the past history in persons with certain illnesses and in healthy persons. As an assessment of the degree of comparability in the interviews, the average length of the interview was 38.2 min in the cases and 36.6 min in the cotrols.

Selection bias was essentially prevented by including all persons who were diagnosed as having bladder cancer during the specified period and by using population controls.

2. Estrogens and Endometrial Cancer

For about 40 years, women with symptoms related to the menopause have been treated with conjugated estrogens. During the menopause, symptoms occur that presumably are related to the decrease in a woman's natural level of estrogens. Treatment with exogenous estrogens has theoretical justification and, more importantly, relieves the symptoms.

However, a component of estrogen therapy has been found to be carcinogenic in rats. To evaluate the possibility that estrogen therapy leads to cancer in humans, a case-control study was done.[5]

The study took place in the membership of the Southern California Kaiser Foundation Health Plan. Between 7/1/70 and 12/31/74, 94 women with endometrial cancer were identified. For each woman with this cancer, two female controls were selected from the list of Plan members. Controls were matched to cases on birth date, zip code, duration of Plan membership, and having an intact uterus. The Health Plan records were searched for information related to estrogen treatment. The searchers did not know whether a given record belonged to a case or to a control. As seen in Table 3.3 almost four times as many cases as controls had been treated with conjugated estrogens.

The reason for the association between estrogen therapy and endometrial cancer has been a source of much discussion. It is unlikely that the association was the result of observation bias, since records were abstracted blindly. Further, for the cases no information obtained 1 year prior to the diagnosis of endometrial cancer was used. Confounding bias by the factors matched upon was not possible, since in the study data they had an equal distribution in cases and in controls. Confounding by other factors was possible. For example, it is possible that women who develop severe menopausal symptoms (and are treated with estrogens) have a higher inherent risk of endometrial cancer than women who have only mild menopausal symptoms.

A major question has been raised on the possibility that selection bias may have led to the association seen. It is argued that women with uterine bleeding who are taking menopausal estrogens are admitted to the hospital and carefully evaluated for endometrial cancer, while women with bleeding who are not taking estrogens are not admitted and not subject to being diagnosed.[6] The argument is that this selection bias leads to a falsely higher proportion of estrogen use among hospitalized women with endometrial cancer.

It has been argued that to control for this presumed selection bias, women with uterine bleeding who do not have endometrial cancer should be used as controls. They would have been submitted to the same diagnostic tests as the women with cancer and thus, if anything, would be subject to the same selection bias as well as the same tests for uterine cancer. This suggestion, however, has been disputed on the grounds of over-matching.[27] If menopausal estrogen therapy causes both endometrial cancer and bleeding for nonspecific reasons, both diagnostic groups would have had more frequent usage of estrogens than other women.

The controversy about possible selection bias or over-matching results primarily because of the nature of case-control studies. Both the exposure and the disease have occurred when the case is enrolled into the study, and the possibility that the diagnosis was influenced by knowledge of the exposure is always present. At the extreme, case-control studies of generally expected associations may inevitably lead to over-estimates of the association.

In reality, however, the extreme rarely happens. Severity of symptoms rather than presence of exposure is the usual criterion for admission to hospital. Persons with severe or acute illnesses are usually admitted to hospital without knowledge of specific exposures.

3. Comment

Case-control studies are occasionally viewed as imperfect or irrelevant simply because the data relate exposure to disease rather than disease to exposure. The "retrospective" view of the exposure-disease association is viewed as unnatural. On theoretical grounds, there is no reason to dismiss case-control studies, for an association between exposure and disease can be detected irrespective of the way the data were collected. Also, empirically, more and more case-control studies are being done.[28]

Of more relevance is the fact that there are always difficulties in the conduct of case-control studies. Confounding, observation, and selection biases are always possible. In the conduct of case-control studies, as in the conduct of cohort studies, efforts must be made to minimize the effects of such biases. Further, since case-control studies are nonexperimental, the interpretation of data resulting from case-control studies must be made with caution.

In the occupational setting, case-control studies have been used less frequently than cohort studies. Usually, there is an interest in which diseases have occurred in a specific occupational group. A cohort study is the natural way to evaluate this interest. However, if one wishes to know which of a number of occupations are associated with a specific disease, a case-control study would be more logical. In such a situation, only fairly common occupations could be evaluated, since a given occupation would not be expected to be present in a large percentage of the cases (or the controls). Case-control studies in the occupational setting, therefore, are most efficient where one or two occupations are common.

F. Cross-Sectional Studies

In a cohort study, persons with and without exposure are selected at the start of the study. In a case-control study, persons with and without disease are selected at the start of the study. In a cross-sectional study, persons are selected irrespective of their exposure or disease status. Exposure and disease are measured essentially at the same point in time. Further, the time sequence between the onset of exposure and the onset of disease cannot be inferred.

The data resulting from a cross-sectional study can be treated as data from a cohort study or as data from a case-control study. That is, disease rates can be compared between exposed and nonexposed groups, or exposure percentages can be compared between diseased and nondiseased groups. The difficulty in evaluating data in a cross-sectional study is to decide whether the exposure led to the disease or the disease led to the exposure.

The fact that data are collected in a cross-sectional manner is not the defining characteristic of a cross-sectional study. The inability to establish the exposure-disease time sequence is the defining characteristic. For example, smoking histories may be obtained on all persons entering a hospital. Disease is diagnosed at essentially the same time. In evaluating the association between lung cancer and cigarette smoking, information is usually available on when the smoking and the disease started. Further, it seems unlikely that the development of lung cancer would lead to cigarette smoking. Also, if one measures aspirin consumption and arthritis, it should be straightforward to establish that the disease (arthritis) led to the exposure (aspirin).

However, consider heart disease and blood cholesterol. It has been felt that high blood cholesterol leads to heart disease. Persons with chest pain may alter their diet and may as a result reduce their levels of blood cholesterol. It is difficult to establish the meaning of cross-sectional data relating blood cholesterol and heart disease.

1. Analgesic Intake and Kidney Disorders

In the late 1960s, in Switzerland, 7311 women were screened for their prevalence of phenacetin use.[29] Phenacetin is an analgesic of potency similar to aspirin. Of these women 623 were found to be using phenacetin at the time of the screening. For comparison purposes, 621 nonusers were selected.

This study was the beginning of a cohort study to measure the incidence rate of kidney disease. However, information was also obtained on kidney disease present at the time of the screening. The data are presented in Table 3.15. Note that while the data in the table give the appearance of selection on exposure or nonexposure, the initial screen was of a larger group of women. The nonexposed group represents a sample of the total group of nonexposed women.

Proteinuria is a sign of kidney disease where protein from the blood serum is excreted into the urine. The rate of proteinuria in the exposed women is twice the rate in those not taking phenacetin. No rate for the total group of women is given. As in a case-control study, where the case-control ratio is usually determined by the investigator, in these data the exposed:not exposed ratio is arbitrary. The rate for the total group, as well as the exposure percentages in diseased and not diseased groups, will vary according to the size of this arbitrary ratio.

In these data, it is unknown which came first, the phenacetin or the proteinuria.

Table 3.15
ASSOCIATION BETWEEN
PROTEINURIA IN WOMEN WITH
AND WITHOUT CURRENT
PHENACETIN USE

Phenacetin use	Proteinuria			
	Yes	No	Total	Rate
Yes	39	584	623	6.3
No	19	602	621	3.1

Phenacetin may lead to kidney disease that causes proteinuria. Conversely, kidney disease with concomitant proteinuria may cause women to take phenacetin for analgesia. The fact of the association is not in question, but its direction is.

As in all other study types, confounding, observation, or selection bias could be present and could account for the association seen.

2. Comment

Cross-sectional studies are relatively uncommon in general epidemiology because an effort usually is made to determine the time sequence of the association being evaluated. However, in occupational settings, cross-sectional data are more likely to be collected.

Data from a preemployment medical examination are usually cross-sectional. For example, a routine questionnaire may have questions on current smoking and current illnesses. Data from a company health insurance plan may be cross-sectional. One knows current work area and current illness. Quite possibly an employee went to his current job because of the rigors of a previous work area. For example, a high rate of heart disease may be found in fork-lift truck drivers. The heart disease might be a result of carbon monoxide exposure, or might be a result of a company policy of placing persons with heart disease in that area. Data resulting from medical screening programs also tend to be cross-sectional.

Cross-sectional data contain no inherent misinformation. However, care is needed in evaluating data to determine whether or not they are indeed cross-sectional. If the time sequence between exposure and disease cannot be determined, an extra degree of caution must be maintained in interpreting any association or nonassociation. The passage of time may be necessary to enable the collection of data in a longitudinal manner to supplement the data collected cross-sectionally.

REFERENCES

1. **Berkson, J.,** Limitation of the application of fourfold table analysis to hospital data, *Biometrics*, 2, 47, 1946.
2. **Roberts, R. S., Spitzer, W. O., Delmore, T., and Sackett, D. L.,** An emperical demonstration of Berkson's bias, *J. Chronic Dis.*, 31, 119, 1978.
3. Boston Collaborative Drug Surveillance Program, Regular aspirin intake and acute myocardial infarction, *Br. Med. J.*, 1, 440, 1974.
4. **Boice, J. D., Jr. and Monson, R. R.,** Breast cancer in women after repeated fluoroscopic examinations of the chest, *J. Nat. Cancer Inst.*, 59, 823, 1977.

5. **Ziel, H. K. and Finkle, W. D.**, Increased risk of endometrial carcinoma among users of conjugated estrogens, *N. Engl. J. Med.*, 293, 1167, 1975.

6. **Horwitz, R. I. and Feinstein, A. R.**, Alternative analytic methods for case-control studies of estrogens and endometrial cancer, *N. Engl. J. Med.*, 299, 1089, 1978.

7. University Group Diabetes Program, A study of the effects of hypoglycemic agents on vascular complications in patients with adult-onset diabetes. II. Mortality results, *Diabetes*, 19 (Suppl. 2), 789, 1970.

8. **Schor, S.**, The University Group Diabetes Program. A statistician looks at the mortality results, *JAMA*, 217, 1671, 1971.

9. **Bradley, R. F., Dolger H., Forsham, P. H., and Seltzer H.**, Settling the UGDP controversy?, *JAMA*, 232, 813, 1975.

10. **Hutter, A. M., Sidel, V. W., Shine, K. I., and DeSanctis, R. W.**, Early hospital discharge after myocardial infarction, *N. Engl. J. Med.*, 288, 1141, 1973.

11. **Silverberg, D., Cancer statistics — 1978**, *Ca*, 28, 17, 1978.

12. **Hoover, R. and Cole, P.**, Population trends in cigarette smoking and bladder cancer, *Am. J. Epidemiol.*, 94, 409, 1971.

13. **Fraumeni, J. F., Jr.**, Cigarette smoking and cancers of the urinary tract: geographic variation in the United States, *J. Nat. Cancer Inst.*, 41, 1205, 1968.

14. **Mason, T. J., McKay, F. W., Hoover, R., Blot, W. J., and Fraumeni, J. F., Jr.**, *Atlas of Cancer Mortality for U.S. Counties: 1950—1969*, DHEW Pub. No. (NIH) 75—780, Department of Health Education and Welfare, Washington, D.C., 1975.

15. **Hoover, R. and Fraumeni, J. F., Jr.**, Cancer mortality in U.S. counties with chemical industries, *Environ. Res.*, 9, 196, 1975.

16. **Page, T., Harris, R. H., and Epstein, S. S.**, Drinking water and cancer mortality in Louisiana, *Science*, 193, 55, 1976.

17. **Yano, K., Rhoads, G. G., and Kagan, A.**, Coffee, alcohol and risk of coronary heart disease among Japanese men living in Hawaii, *N. Engl. J. Med.*, 297, 405, 1977.

18. **Heinonen, O. P., Slone, D., and Shapiro, S.**, *Birth Defects and Drugs in Pregnancy*, Publishing Sciences Group, Littleton, Mass., 1977.

19. **Doll, R. and Peto, R.**, Mortality in relation to smoking: 20 years' observations on male British doctors, *Br. Med. J.*, 2, 1525, 1976.

20. **Hammond, E. C.**, Smoking in relation to the death rates of one million men and women, *Nat. Cancer Inst. Monogr.*, No. 19, 127, 1966.

21. **Kahn, H. A.**, The Dorn study of smoking and mortality among U.S. veterans: report on eight and one-half years of observations, *Nat. Cancer Inst. Monogr.*, No. 19, 1, 1966.

22. **Lloyd, J. W. and Ciocco, A.**, Long-term mortality study of steelworkers. I. Methodology, *J. Occup. Med.*, 11, 299, 1969.

23. **Redmond, C. K., Smith, E. M., Lloyd, J. W., and Rush, H. W.**, Long-term mortality study of steelworkers. III. Follow-up, *J. Occup. Med.*, 11, 513, 1969.

24. **Redmond, C. K., Strobino, B. R., and Cypess R. H.**, Cancer experience among coke by-product workers, *Ann. N.Y. Acad. Sci.*, 271, 102, 1976.

25. **Boice, J. D., Jr.**, Follow-up methods to trace women treated for pulmonary tuberculosis, *Am. J. Epidemiol.*, 107, 127, 1978.

26. **Cole, P., Monson, R. R., Haning, H., and Friedell, G. H.**, Smoking and cancer of the lower urinary tract, *N. Engl. J. Med.*, 284, 129, 1971.

27. **Hutchison, G. B. and Rothman, K. R.**, Correcting a bias?, *N. Engl. J. Med.*, 299, 1129, 1978.

28. **Cole, P., The evolving case-control study**, *J. Chronic Dis.*, 32, 15, 1979.

29. **Dubach, U. C., Levy, P. S., and Mueller, A.**, Relationships between regular analgesic intake and urorenal disorders in a working female population of Switzerland. I. Initial results (1968). *Am. J. Epidemiol.*, 93, 425, 1971.

Chapter 4
THE ANALYSIS OF EPIDEMIOLOGIC DATA

I. INTRODUCTION

Data consist of numbers. The data contain no information as to their source. It follows that similar analyses can be performed on data from different sources.

In Chapter 2, the two basic types of rates in epidemiology are described: incidence rates and prevalence rates. (An attack rate has the units of a prevalence rate.) Each is used to measure the occurrence of disease in a population; the comparison of two or more rates of the same type is the basic procedure in data analysis. In the search for causes of disease, an epidemiologist may compare the incidence rate in an exposed group to the incidence rate in a nonexposed group. In the search for cures of disease, an epidemiologist may compare the cure rate in a treated group to the cure rate in a nontreated group. In this context the cure rate is an example of an attack rate.

The basic characteristic of incidence-type rates is that time is part of the units: cases/population/time. For example, a mortality rate may be deaths/1000 persons/year. In contrast, prevalence-type rates are simply cases per population; a cure rate may be persons cured/100 persons treated.

In the analysis of incidence-type rates or prevalence-type rates, there are some similarities and some differences. Crudely, two incidence rates can be compared using the rate ratio or the rate difference; these ratios also can be used in comparing two attack rates. In the control of confounding, direct and indirect standardization procedures may be used with either incidence rates or prevalence rates.

However, there are also differences in the analysis of data based on different types of rates. Some of these differences relate to whether rates of two subsets of a population are being compared (internal comparison) or rates are being compared between two populations (external comparison). Also, within prevalence-type data, different analyses are done depending upon whether the ratio of diseased to nondiseased persons is arbitrarily set by the investigator or not. These situations will be considered separately.

The basic goal of data is to relate two rates so that any association between cause and effect in the data reflects as closely as possible the true association in the population under study. However, since this true association will never be known with precision, in analyzing data an epidemiologist is limited to evaluating associations only within the data. The basic exercise in the analysis of epidemiologic data is the search for and control of confounding bias. If a crude association is seen between an exposure and a disease, a search must be made for third factors that may be responsible for the association. The end result is an adjusted or standardized rate ratio.

A secondary goal in data analysis is to provide a measure of the stability of any association seen. This measure is provided by tests of statistical significance or by confidence intervals. Any association may be stable or unstable, depending upon the magnitude of the association and the amount of data upon which the association is based.

II. BASIC COMPARISONS WITHIN EPIDEMIOLOGIC DATA

As discussed in Chapter 2, the rate ratio (relative risk, risk ratio) is the basic measure of association in epidemiologic data. In judging whether an association is likely to be causal, the rate ratio is the measure usually considered. The rate difference (attributable risk, risk difference) is a measure of the excess rate of disease among the exposed.

Another measure occasionally used is the "population rate difference" (population attributable risk).[1] This is the difference between the disease rate in the total population and that in the non-exposed. The rate difference may be expressed as a percentage of the rate among the exposed, and the population rate difference may be expressed as a percentage of the rate among the total population.

The population rate difference percentage (PRDP) is an estimate of the percentage of disease among the total population that is due to the exposure, assuming that the association is causal. While this appears to be a useful measure, it must be used with caution. If the PRDP is computed for a number of variables in a given set of data, the individual PRDPs may add up to over 100%. This results because not all positive associations are causal, because negative PRDPs usually are not computed, and because confounding is not always controlled. Therefore, while the PRDP has the appearance of general meaning, its true value is limited.

The most basic form of displaying epidemiologic data is in a fourfold or two by two table. Data are presented for disease (yes, no) and exposure (yes, no). If there are more than two categories of exposure (or of disease) data are displayed in a 2 × n table, where "n" is the number of categories of exposure (or of disease). Finally, with multiple categories of exposure and of disease, data are displayed in a n × n table.

A. Two by Two Tables
1. Prevalence-Type Data

Prevalence-type data are data in which the denominator of a rate is persons. Prevalence rates and attack rates are the usual examples of such data. Prevalence rates usually are measured in cross-sectional studies. Attack rates usually are measured in experimental or prospective cohort studies.

In Table 4.1, the basic layout for prevalence-type data is presented. The data are entered into the usual fourfold table. Attack or prevalence rates are computed among the exposed and the nonexposed. They may be related using the rate ratio or the rate difference. Computation of the population rate difference and the PRDP may be carried out. These are all straight-forward, definitional relationships.

One way to assess the stability of the rate ratio is by inspection. If the size of "a" is small, say less than five, it is intuitively obvious that the exchange of one or two persons between "a" and "c" will result in a large alteration in the size of the rate ratio. Clearly, if the study were repeated, the rate ratio could be much smaller or much larger. The intuitive method of assessing stability has much to offer.

A measure of stability of the rate ratio can also be computed. In order to do so, one must estimate both the "expected value of a" or "E(a)" and the "variance of a" or "V(a)". E(a) is the size "a" would be if there were no association between exposure and disease. In this event, the rate of disease among the exposed, the rate of disease among the nonexposed, and the rate of disease among the total population would be equal. V(a) is a statistical formula based on the number of persons in the margins of the table. In general, the larger the total number in the study is, the smaller is the variance of "a".

Chi-square is a classic test of stability.[2] It relates the square of the difference between "a" and E(a) to V(a). In a two by two table, X^2 has one degree of freedom. By looking in a table of X^2, one can obtain the "p-value" for a given X^2 and a given number of degrees of freedom.[3] As a measure of stability, the p-value indicates the likelihood that, if the study were repeated a number of times, a rate ratio as large as or larger than that obtained would occur, given no true association between exposure and disease. This assumes that the data are unbiased.

Table 4.1
BASIC ANALYSIS OF PREVALENCE-TYPE DATA

| Exposure | Disease | | Total | Rate |
	Yes	No		
Yes	a	b	a + b	a/(a + b)
No	c	d	c + d	c/(c + d)
Total	a + c	b + d	N	(a + c)/N

1.   Measures of association
 a.   Rate ratio (RR) = $a/(a + b) \div c/(c + d)$
 b.   Rate difference (RD) = $a/(a + b) - c/(c + d)$
 c.   Population rate difference (PRD) = $(a + c)/N - c/(c + d)$
 d.   Population rate difference percent (PRDP) = $100 \times PRD/(a + c)/N$

2.   Measure of stability
 a.   Expected value of "a", given no association between exposure and disease
    $[E(a)] = (a + b)(a + c)/N$
 b.   Variance of "a" $[V(a)] = [(a + c)(b + d)(a + b)(c + d)]/N^2(N - 1)$
 c.   Chi-square $(X^2_1) = [a - E(a)]^2/V(a)$
 d.   95% Confidence interval[4]
    upper limit = $RR \exp(1 + 1.96/X)$
    lower limit = $RR \exp(1 - 1.96/X)$ (exp = exponent)

A confidence interval is a variation of a p-value.[4] If a number of 95% confidence intervals are computed, the true rate ratio will be expected to lie within 95% of the intervals, assuming that the data are not biased. For a given confidence interval, however, the true rate ratio either is in or out; it is unknown which is the case.

Epidemiologists differ in their proclivity to compute measures of stability on epidemiologic data. In general, if a measure is to be computed, the confidence interval is preferable. However, a p-value or a confidence interval provide no measure of the meaning of an association. Unfortunately, the term "statistically significant" frequently is taken to mean "causally associated". As a result, the interpretation of data may become reduced to the computation of a number. I prefer to think of p-values and confidence limits as simply measures of stability. Since stability can be roughly assessed by inspection, formal computation of one or two numbers is not always necessary or even advisable.

The formulas in Tables 4.1 to 4.3 show *how* to compute chi-squares and confidence intervals. *Whether* they should be computed is another matter. As the numbers of persons in the study become smaller, these formulas become increasingly inaccurate in the statistical sense. Further, the confidence interval becomes so wide as to have little meaning. I see little utility to the computation of a measure of stability if "a" is less than five. With larger numbers, judgment is needed as to the value of a measure of stability. If there are known to be sources of bias that may or may not be controllable, a p-value or confidence interval based on the crude (biased) (confounded) data has little meaning, just as does the rate ratio.

On occasion, data as those in Table 4.1 come from a study in which the ratio of exposed to nonexposed is arbitrarily set by the investigator. In this situation, unless the true ratio of exposed to nonexposed in the population can be determined, the quantity (a + c)/N has no meaning. Also, the population rate difference and the PRDP

Table 4.2
BASIC ANALYSIS OF INCIDENCE-TYPE DATA

Disease

Exposure	Yes	No	Person-years	Rate
Yes	a	—	PYRSe	a/PYRSe
No	c	—	PYRSo	c/PYRSo
Total	a + c	—	PYRSt	(a + c)/PYRSt

1. Measures of association
    a. Rate ratio (RR) = a/PYRSe ÷ c/PYRSo
    b. Rate difference (RD) = a/PYRSe − c/PYRSo
    c. Population rate difference (PRD) = (a + c)/PYRSt − c/PYRSo
    d. Population rate difference percent PRDP = $100 \times$ PRD/(a + c)/ PYRst

2. Measure of stability
    a. Expected value of "a", given no association between exposure and disease [E(a)] = PYRSe (a + c)/PYRSt
    b. Variance of "a", assuming a is small relative to PYRSe [V(a)] = E(a) (Poisson assumption)
    c. Chi-square (X^2_1) = $[a - E(a)]^2/V(a)$
    d. 95% Confidence interval
        upper limit = RR exp (1 + 1.96/X)
        lower limit = RR exp (1 − 1.96/X) (exp = exponent)

are inaccurate. However, the rate ratio, the rate difference, and the measures of stability may all be computed in the usual manner.

Example — Consider the data in Study 1 in Table 2.2, Chapter 2. The rate ratio is $10.5 \div 6.4 = 1.6$. The rate difference is $10.5 - 6.4 = 4.1/100$. The population rate difference is $6.5 - 6.4 = 0.1/100$. The PRDP is $0.1/100 \div 6.5/100 = 1.5\%$. This means that if the association between epilepsy and malformations is causal, epilepsy has caused 1.5% of the malformations in this population.

The expected value of "a" [E(a)], is $3248 \times 305/50,282 = 19.7$. The variance of "a" = $(3248)(47,034)(305)(49,977)/(50,282)(50,282)(50,281) = 18$. Chi-square = $[32 - 19.7]^2/18 = 8.4$. The upper 95% confidence limit is 1.6 exp $(1 + 1.96/\sqrt{8.4}) = 1.6^{(1.68)} = 2.2$. The lower 95% confidence limit is 1.6 exp $(1 - 1.96/\sqrt{8.4}) = 1.6^{(0.32)} = 1.2$.

2. Incidence-Type Data

Incidence-type data are data in which the denominator of a rate is person-years. Incidence rates and mortality rates are the usual example of such data. These rates usually are measured in experimental or in cohort studies.

In Table 4.2, the basic data layout for incidence-type data is presented. The usual fourfold table is modified in that rather than total number of exposed, nonexposed, and all persons in the denominators of the rates, person-years are used. Computation of the measures of association is similar to the computations on prevalence-type data. As in Table 4.1, if the ratio of exposed to nonexposed is arbitrarily set by the investigator, the total incidence rate, the population rate difference and the PRDP have no inherent meaning.

As with prevalence-type data, the computation of a measure of stability is not advisable when the number of persons with disease is small. In estimating the variance of "a", the Poisson assumption holds only when "a" is small relative to PYRSe, (or more generally, "a + c" is small relative to PYRSt). With this assumption, the computations of X^2 and the 95% confidence interval are similar to those used for prevalence-type data.

In the computation of person-years, one person who is followed for 10 years contributes the same number as ten persons followed for 1 year. While on theoretical grounds objections can be raised to this equality, I am not aware of any instances where errors in interpretation have arisen.

Example — Consider the data in Table 2.6. The rate ratio based on incidence rates is $1.5 \div 6.7 = 0.22$. The rate difference is $1.5/1000/month - 6.7/1000/month = -5.2/1000/month$. The negative rate difference means that, if the association is causal, the exposure prevents the disease. The population rate difference is $4.1 - 6.7 = -2.6/1000/month$. The PRDP is $-2.6/1000/month \div 6.7/1000/month = -39\%$. In this example of a vaccine preventing disease, the population risk difference percent is thought of as the percent of potential disease prevented by the exposure;[5] the potential rate in the total population is $6.7/1000/month$. The expected value of "a" is the person-months among the exposed times the rate of disease in the total population. This works out to 100,000 person months $\times 4.1/1000/month = 410$. $X^2 = (149 - 410)^2/410 = 166$. The lower 95% confidence limit is $0.22 \exp (1 + 1.96/\sqrt{166}) = 0.22^{1.15} = 0.18$. The upper 95% confidence limit is $0.22 \exp (1 - 1.96/\sqrt{166}) = 0.22^{0.85} = 0.28$. The formulas for the upper and lower limits are reversed because the rate ratio is less than 1.0. Because the rate ratio is based on relatively large numbers of persons, the confidence interval is narrow.

3. Case-Control Data

In experimental, cohort and cross-sectional studies, meaningful rates of disease can be computed. Also, in case control studies where all cases in a defined population are identified, rates of disease can be computed. In most case-control studies, however, this is not possible. The ratio of persons with and without disease is usually set by the investigator. As a result, the rate of disease among the exposed (or among the nonexposed) is completely arbitrary. For example, in a case-control study with one control per case, the rate of disease in the persons studied is 50/100.

However, this is only a minor problem. If the rate of disease is rare in the general population, the odds ratio as defined in Table 4.3 is a good estimate of the rate ratio.[6] Further, if the cases are new (incident) cases of disease rather than old or prevalent cases, the odds ratio is equivalent to the rate ratio.[4] Finally, even if neither of these conditions hold, the odds ratio itself is a measure that can be interpreted essentially the same as the rate ratio.

Unless all new cases in a defined population are ascertained over some period, the absolute sizes of the rate difference and the population rate difference are not measurable. However, the PRDP may be approximated.[7] As seen in Table 4.3, the measures of stability used in the analysis of data from case-control studies are the same as those used in the analysis of prevalence-type data. The margins of the table are used in these computations.

Example — Consider the data in Study two in Table 2.2. The odds ratio is $(8) (2782)/(2)(2776) = 4.0$. The PRDP is $[(4 - 1)/4] \times 100 = 75\%$. The expected value of "a" [E(a)] is $10 \times 2784/5568 = 5.0$. The variance of "a" $= (2784)(2784)(5558)(10)/(5568)(5568)(5567) = 2.5$. $X^2 = [8 - 5.0]^2/2.5 = 3.6$. The upper 95% confidence limit $= 4.0 \exp (1 + 1.96/\sqrt{3.6}) = 4^{2.0} = 16.0$. The lower 95% confidence limit $= 4 \exp (1 - 1.96/\sqrt{3.6}) = 4^{-0.03} = 0.96$. Even though the odds ratio is high, the confidence interval is wide because of the small number of mothers with epilepsy and phenytoin use.

Table 4.3
BASIC ANALYSIS OF
CASE-CONTROL
DATA

	Disease	
Exposure	Yes	No
Yes	a	b
No	c	d
Total	a + c	d + d

1. Measures of association
   a. Rate ratio (RR) $\doteq$ odds ratio (OR) = ad/bc
   b. Rate difference (RD); population rate difference (PRD): usually not known
   c. Population rate difference percent (PRDP) = $100 \times (OR - 1)/OR$

2. Measure of stability — see Table 1

B. Two by N Tables

A 2 by N table is simply a variant of a 2 × 2 table (Table 4.4). Analogous computations for rate ratios and risk differences can be made. The rate of disease in one level of exposure is chosen arbitrarily as the rate to which the other rates in the table are compared. If the data in Table 4.4 came from a case-control study with an arbitrary ratio of cases to controls, the odds ratio for the nonexposed would be arbitrarily set at 1.0. The odds ratio for the medium exposure group would be cf/de, and that for the high exposure group would be af/be.

In computing X^2, the sum of the quantity $(O - E)^2/E$ for each cell is obtained.[2] As the number of cells increases, so does the number of degrees of freedom. The X^2 with two degrees of freedom provides a measure of the overall variation within the table.

Data from a 2 × N table can be converted into a variety of 2 × 2 tables. From the data in Table 4.4, six 2 × 2 tables could be constructed:

1. High + medium vs. none
2. High + none vs. medium
3. Medium + none vs. high
4. High vs. none
5. Medium vs. none
6. High vs. medium

Six rate ratios, X^2 and confidence intervals could be computed.

Whether such rearrangement of data and computation of many rate ratios and p-values are proper is a subject of discussion among epidemiologists and statisticians. Certainly, the computations can be done and the measurements made. However, the interpretation of the results of such computations must be even more cautious than

Table 4.4
DATA IN A 2 BY N TABLE

Exposure	Disease			
	Yes	No	Total	Rate
High	a	b	a + b	a/a + b)
Medium	c	d	c + d	c/(c + d)
None	e	f	e + f	e/(e + f)
Total	a + c + e	b + d + f	N	

1. Measure of association

   Rate ratio (high)   =   a/(a + b) ÷ e/(e + f)
   Rate ratio (medium)   =   c/(c + d) ÷ e/(e + f)
   Rate ratio (none)   =   e/(e + f) ÷ e/(e + f) = 1.0

2. Measure of stability

   O   = observed number in each cell (a, b, c, d, e, or f)
   E   = expected number in each cell
         E(a) = (a + b)(a + c + e)/N, and so on
   X^2_n = $\Sigma[(O - E)^2/E]$
   Σ = sum of
         n = degrees of freedom = $(r - 1) \times (c - 1)$
         r = number of rows
         c = number of columns
         n = 2 in this example

Table 4.5
DATA IN AN N × N TABLE

Exposure	Disease			
	Severe	Moderate	None	Total
High	a	b	c	a + b + c
Medium	d	e	f	d + e + f
Low	g	h	i	g + h + i
Total	a + d + g	b + e + h	c + f + i	N

usual. Chance associations are likely in all data, and the likelihood is great that many associations seen when data are rearranged are simply due to chance. No statistical test can distinguish between chance and causal associations.

C. N by N Tables

In Table 4.5, three levels of exposure and three levels of disease are presented. It can be seen that the analysis of such data has the potential to become complicated. Yet such tables form the basic output of many cross-tabulations performed under packaged programs such as SPSS.[8]

Rather than computing a number of rate ratios on the data in this form, it frequently is useful to combine strata. For example, if the rates of disease among the low and medium exposure groups are similar, the data can be degraded into a 2 × 3 table.

Such combining of strata in complex tables is a basic procedure to be used in describing the results of a study. The more simply the data can be presented, the better. However, in my opinion, it is improper to compute a measure of stability after such

Table 4.6
ASSOCIATION OF SELECTED CHARACTERISTICS OF PREGNANCY WITH PHENYTOIN USAGE AND WITH CONGENITAL MALFORMATIONS

Characteristic	Phenytoin use		Rate ratio of congenital malformations[a]
	Yes	No	
Birthweight < 2500 g	13.3	11.3	2.0
Black ethnic group	37.8	47.8	1.6
Mother's age 35 or above	12.2	7.2	1.4
Bleeding during pregnancy	33.7	26.0	1.0
Mother's cigarette smoking	36.7	46.2	1.0
Prenatal X-ray exposure	35.7	22.5	1.0

[a]   Rate of malformation in children with characteristic divided by rate of malformation in children without characteristic.

collapsing of data. Part of the reason for the stability of the data is the fact that the investigator looked at the data and made judicious combinations. No longer can the data be used to measure the likelihood of random processes. Whereas the rate ratio obtained from collapsed data is a useful measure of the association seen *in that study,* a p-value or confidence limit based on collapsed data partially reflects the actions of the investigator.

If unexpected associations are found in any data, simple or complex, they should be reported. If complicated data can be simplified, it should be done. However, interpretation of such associations must rely heavily on data obtained under independent circumstances and hardly at all on measures of stability from the initial study.

III. ASSESSMENT OF COMPARABILITY

In the analysis of all epidemiologic data, an initial step is to decide which factors are likely to be confounding. If a crude association is seen between an exposure and a disease (rate ratio $\neq$ 1.0), the association could be due to confounding bias if there is some third factor that is both an independent cause of the disease and is associated with the exposure. Also, if no association between an exposure and a disease is seen, (rate ratio = 1.0), a true causal association could be masked because of negative confounding: another cause of the disease is more common among the nonexposed than among the exposed.

To assess the possibility of confounding, the first step is to measure the association of the exposure with the third factor and of the disease with the third factor. If the factor can be shown *not* to be associated either with the exposure *or* the disease, it cannot be confounding. For example, consider the data in Table 4.6. These data were obtained in a preliminary evaluation of the association between phenytoin (diphenyl-hydantoin) and birth defects.[9] Crudely, birth defects were 2.5 times more common in children born to women who took phenytoin relative to children born to women who did not take phenytoin.

The factors in the top half of the Table needed to be controlled, because each was associated both with phenytoin use and congenital malformations. The association of low birth weight with phenytoin use is very weak, and very little confounding could be introduced. The association of mother's age with the rate ratio of congenital malformations is also very weak. However, in theory at least, considerable confounding could be introduced by a number of weak confounding factors acting in the same direction. In practice, there usually are negative confounding factors that tend to counter-balance those that are positively confounding. Black ethnicity is a negative confounder; it is negatively associated with phenytoin use and positively associated with congenital malformations. Control for black ethnicity will, if anything, increase the association between birth defects and phenytoin use.

The factors in the bottom half of the Table are not associated with congenital malformations. Therefore, no matter how strongly these factors are associated with phenytoin use, they cannot be confounding. Also, factors associated with congenital malformations but not associated with phenytoin use cannot be confounding.

In assessing whether a factor is likely to be confounding, one does not compute p-values or confidence intervals. The decision as to whether a third factor is likely to be confounding is totally a matter of judgment. If there is any question as to the possibility of confounding, a standardized rate ratio should be computed and compared to the crude rate ratio.

Judgement as to the likelihood of confounding is partially a matter of experience. However, guidelines can be given. If the crude rate ratio between an exposure and a disease is high, say 5.0, and the measure of association between a third factor and either the exposure or the disease is low, say less than 2.0, very little confounding could be introduced by the third factor. At worst, assuming there is complete correlation beteen the factor and the exposure, such correlation could lead only to a rate ratio of 2.0 between the exposure and the disease. However, if a third factor is strongly associated with an exposure (say RR = 10) and moderately associated with the disease (say RR = 3) an association between the exposure and the disease of RR = 2 could readily be due to confounding.

In most epidemiologic data, confounding bias can not be shown to account for many associations. Most characteristics of humans are only weakly associated both with other factors and with diseases. Certainly there are exceptions, for example, between drugs and medical conditions for which they are prescribed. Certainly the search for and control of confounding bias is a necessary part of all epidemiologic studies. But it is surprising that frequently the crude association seen between exposure and disease turns out to be the overall best measure of the association.

In this discussion of comparability, no confounding by a factor is possible unless the factor is (crudely) associated both with the exposure and the disease. While in general this is true, there can be data that do not conform. There may be two or more factors that, while not crudely associated with exposure and disease, are associated when compared jointly. While I am not aware of any serious misinterpretation in epidemiologic studies because of a failure to seek out such situations, the possibility must be kept in mind. If there is serious concern about possible interaction, all factors involved should be controlled, possibly using a multivariate technique (q.v.).

Also, a third factor may be an *effect modifier* rather than a confounder. Effect modification means that the rate ratio (or odds ratio) differ across strata of a third factor. Small differences are usual simply because of probabilistic nature of biologic data. On occasion, however, an association may be positive in one stratum of a population and negative in a second.

Consider the data in Table 4.7. These data were obtained in a study in which persons with bladder cancer were asked about their past use of artificial sweeteners.[10] In the crude data, the odds ratio of bladder cancer associated with the use of artificial sweeteners was $(91)(555)/(541)(77) = 1.2$. However, when the data were stratified according

Table 4.7
ASSOCIATION BETWEEN THE USE OF ARTIFICIAL SWEETENERS AND BLADDER CANCER IN MEN AND WOMEN

	Men				Women	
	Bladder cancer				Bladder cancer	
Use of artificial sweeteners	Yes	No		Use of artificial sweeteners	Yes	No
Yes	73	47		Yes	18	30
No	407	433		No	134	122
Total	480	480		Total	152	152

OR = (73)(433)/(407)(47) = 1.65   OR = (18)(122)/(134)(30) = 0.55

to sex, the odds ratio in men was 1.65 and in women was 0.55. In such a situation, computation of a standardized odds ratio is of questionable value. If these data reflect causal associations (and that is questionable), artificial sweeteners appear to cause bladder cancer in men and to prevent bladder cancer in women. Clearly, the interpretation of these data is difficult.

IV. THE CONTROL OF CONFOUNDING

A. Standardization of Rates
A basic technique in data analysis is the standardization of rates. One purpose of standardization is the control of confounding. If two populations have different age distributions, age will be confounding if disease rates differ by age. If two populations have different occupational distributions, occupation will be confounding if disease rates differ by occupation. However, if in a body of data a disease has the same rate in different age groups, age is not confounding.

Two general types of standardization are in common use: direct and indirect. Each type has strengths and weaknesses; no type is best in all circumstances. Each type may be used with incidence-type data or with prevalence-type data.

1. Direct Standardization
Consider the data in Table 4.8. Suppose that a disease that is more prevalent in older ages exists in a population. Within the population there are three groups of differing age distributions but whose age-specific disease rates are the same. Since Group A is older than Groups B and C, the crude rate of disease in Group A is the highest. This higher rate occurs only because the persons in Group A are older and not because Group A is more "dangerous". Relative to Group C, the crude rate ratio of disease in Group A is 9.2/6.8 = 1.35.

In this example, age is confounding. By standardizing or adjusting for age, the confounding can be controlled. A standardized rate ratio can be computed that shows the relation between disease and being a member of Group A, B, or C independent of age.

Table 4.8
AN EXAMPLE OF CONFOUNDING BY AGE

Age	Rate of disease	Group A		Group B		Group C	
		Total number	Number with disease	Total number	Number with disease	Total number	Number with disease
<45	4/100	200	8	300	12	500	20
45—54	8/100	300	24	400	32	300	24
≥55	12/100	500	60	300	36	200	24
	Total	1000	92	1000	80	1000	68
Crude rate		9.2/100		8.0/100		6.8/100	

The reason that the crude rate of disease in Group A is high is that a higher percentage of Group A is aged 55 and above. The crude rate of 9.2 is a function of both the age-specific rates and the numbers in each age group. These numbers are termed *weights*. The age-specific rates in Groups A, B, and C are equal; the age-specific weights differ. Since the crude rate in each group is a *weighted average* of the age-specific rates, Group A will have the highest crude rate and Group C will have the lowest.

In Table 4.8 the weights are Group A — 2:3:5, Group B — 3:4:3, Group C — 5:3:2. In order to compute a directly-standardized rate of disease in each group, one assigns arbitrarily the same weights to each group. A conventional practice is to use the weights of the total population; in this example the weights are 10:10:10 or 1:1:1. Another common practice is to use the weights of one of the groups, say 2:3:5.

In Table 4.9, the computation of the crude rates is illustrated in Example 1. First, the number of persons with disease in each age stratum is computed. The sum of these age-specific numbers divided by the total number in each group is the crude rate. Note that this total number is the sum of the weights (e.g., Group A = 1000 = 200 + 300 + 500).

In Example 2, a directly-standardized weighted average of the age-specific rates is computed using weights of 1:1:1. Again, first the number of persons with disease in each stratum is calculated. In Group A it is [0.04 + 0.08 + 0.12] = 0.24. Next, this number is divided by the sum of the weights: 0.24 ÷ 3 = 8/100. Since the weights are the same in Group A, B, and C, the age-standardized rates are the same. In Example 2 it may be somewhat disconcerting to use such small weights. However, the absolute size of the weights is completely arbitrary, since all that is being done is a relative weighting of rates.

In Example 2 the rate is computed by dividing the total number of persons with disease (0.24) by the sum of the weights (3). In Example 3 an alternate computational method is used. Since, proportionally, the weights for each group must be equal, the sum can be arbitrarily set at 1.0. In Example 3 the same relative weights as for Group A in Example 1 are used. The directly-standardized rate then is the same as the crude rate for Group A.

As seen in Table 4.9, there is no absolute meaning in the size of a standardized rate. The only meaning is how it relates to some other rate that has been standardized using the same weights. We have divided by the sum of the weights in order to have the standardized rates be roughly the same size as the crude rates. However, if in Example 2 we did not divide by three, the age-standardized rates in Groups A, B, and C would each be 24/100. The ratio of these rates is still 1:1:1.

Table 4.9
EXAMPLES OF DIRECT STANDARDIZATION OF DATA IN
TABLE 4.8

Example 1. Computation of crude rates

Group A: [200(4/100) + 300(8/100) + 500(12/100)] ÷ 1000 = 9.2/100
Group B: [300(4/100) + 400(8/100) + 300(12/100)] ÷ 1000 = 8.0/100
Group C: [500(4/100) + 300(8/100) + 200(12/100)] ÷ 1000 = 6.8/100

Example 2. Computation of standardized rates with 1:1:1 weights

Group A: [1(4/100) + 1(8/100) + 1(12/100)] ÷ 3 = 8/100
Group B: [1(4/100) + 1(8/100) + 1(12/100)] ÷ 3 = 8/100
Group C: [1(4/100) + 1(8/100) + 1(12/100)] ÷ 3 = 8/100

Example 3. Computation of standardized rates with 0.2: 0.3: 0.5 weights

Group A: [0.2(4/100) + 0.3(8/100) + 0.5(12/100)] ÷ 1 = 9.2/100
Group B: [0.2(4/100) + 0.3(8/100) + 0.5(12/100)] ÷ 1 = 9.2/100
Group C: [0.2(4/100) + 0.3(8/100) + 0.5(12/100)] ÷ 1 = 9.2/100

Direct standardization may readily be adapted to the control of two or more variables. Suppose that in addition to age we wished to control for sex. Instead of three age-specific groups there would be six sex-age-specific groups. The computations would be the same.

The major difficulty with direct standardization lies in its instability when the number of strata is large relative to the number of persons in the numerator of the stratum-specific rates. Suppose that in Table 4.9 we wished to standardize for five age, two sex, two race, and three smoking groups. There would be $5 \times 2 \times 2 \times 3 = 60$ potential strata instead of the three age strata used. Since in Group C there were only 68 persons with the disease, some strata would probably have no persons with the disease (rate = 0). In others the rate might be very high, even 1/1. The stratum-specific rates would therefore be unstable. Depending upon the distribution of weights used, a standardized rate might be very low or very high. Simply changing the distribution of weights could greatly change the standardized rate.

In general terms, a crude rate (R) is:

$$R = D/P \qquad\qquad (4.1)$$

where D is the number with the disease and P is the number in the population. A directly standardized rate is:[11,12]

$$R' = \frac{\Sigma W_i r_i}{\Sigma W_i} \qquad\qquad (4.2)$$

where W_i is the stratum-specific weight and r_i is the stratum specific rate. (Σ means sum of).

The standardized (or crude) rate is a measure of disease frequency. The stability of the measure is given by the *Standard Error* (SE):[12]

$$SE = \sqrt{\frac{\Sigma(W_i^2 r_i (1 - r_i) w_i)}{(\Sigma W_i)^2}} \qquad\qquad (4.3)$$

where Wi and ri are as in Equation 4.2 and wi is the group-stratum specific number of persons. The *variance* is the square of the SE.

To compare two age-standardized rates, a common measure of association is the rate ratio: one rate divided by the second. To measure the stability of the rate ratio, one method is to subtract two SE from the higher rate (R1) and add two SE to the lower rate (R2). If $(R1 - 2SE_{R1})$ is higher than $(R2 + 2SE_{R2})$, the two age-adjusted rates differ significantly at less than the 5% level. Alternatively, the difference between the two rates and the SE of the difference can be computed.[12]

Note that neither the rate ratio nor the SE convey any information as to the *meaning* of the association. A high rate ratio may be due to cause, chance, or bias just as can a low rate ratio. Likewise, cause, chance, or bias can produce an association that is "statistically significant". Further, an association that is not significant may nevertheless reflect the causal effects of some factor. The interpretation of data must not rely only on the results of data analysis.

2. Indirect Standardization

Consider again the data in Table 4.8. Suppose that the age-specific rates in each of the three groups were not known, but only the age distributions and the total number with disease in each group. It can be seen that the total number in Group A (92) is higher than the number in Group C (68). Also, the persons in Group A are older than those in Group C. An alternate way to control for this age difference is to compute the number of cases of disease expected in each group on the basis of the overall age-specific rates in the total population. Rather than using standard *weights*, one uses standard *rates*.

In Table 4.10 the number of cases of disease expected in each group is computed by multiplying the age-specific rates for the total population times the number of persons in each age stratum. The number actually observed is divided by the number expected on the basis of this computation. As can be seen, the observed and expected numbers are equal, showing that after correction for age, the occurrence of disease in the three groups is the same.

The analysis illustrated in Table 4.10 led to the proper conclusion because the standard rates used were the same as the actual rates in each of the groups. Suppose that standard rates of 8/100, 16/100, and 24/100 were used. The observed/expected ratios then would be: Group A — 92/184, Group B — 80/160, Group C—68/136. Again, each group would be shown to be similar in that, relative to the population from which the standard rates were drawn, each had 50% of the expected disease occurrence.

Suppose, however, that the standard rates were 4/100, 3/100, and 2/100. The observed/expected numbers would now be: Group A — 92/27 = 3.4, Group B — 80/30 = 2.7, and Group C — 68/33 = 2.1. Here Group A would appear to have over 50% more disease than Group C. Note that, relative to the population from which the standard rates were taken, each of the above ratios is correct. Group C should have a crude rate closer to that of the outside population because 50% of its members are less than 45 and the rates at age 45 are 4/100, as in the standard population. Only 20% of Group A are aged less than 45.

This example illustrates a difficulty that may arise when two or more groups are to be compared using indirect standardization. If the weights of the groups differ, the groups may appear to differ if indirect standardization is used whereas there is no difference when compared directly.

3. Comment

The difficulties with direct standardization tend to be practical. Frequently, in data

Table 4.10
AN EXAMPLE OF INDIRECT STANDARDIZATION OF
DATA IN TABLE 4.8

Group A: Expected number = (4/100)(200) + (8/100)(300) + (12/100)(500) = 92.0
Observed/expected = 92/92.0
Group B: Expected number = (4/100)(300) + (8/100)(400) + (12/100)(300) = 80.0
Observed/expected = 80/80.0
Group C: Expected number = (4/100)(500) + (8/100)(300) + (12/100)(200) = 68.0
Observed/expected = 68/68.0

analysis, an epidemiologist wishes to compare disease rates in several groups to the rates in some large outside population. If, for example, age, sex, and race are to be controlled, the age-sex-race group specific rates may be based on small numbers and may be quite unstable. However, the age-sex-race specific rates in the outside population are based on much larger numbers and are stable. A comparison of observed to expected numbers is much more practical.

The difficulties with indirect standardization tend to be theoretical. It is uncommon for age or other distributions within groups being compared to differ greatly. Fairly extreme mal-distributions are needed for indirect standardization to give misleading results.

However, if stable rates in specific strata are present in data, direct standardization is preferable. The same weights are used for each group and no question exists as to the meaning of the standardized comparison. If only two groups are being compared to each other, either direct or indirect standardization may be used.

B. Standardization of Measures of Association
1. Standardized Rate Ratios

The standardization of rate ratios is simply an extension of the standardization of rates. If one wishes to standardize rate ratios obtained in studies where rates are measured, the standardized rate ratio (SRR) is the ratio of two standardized rates as computed from Formula 4.2. This holds true for either incidence-type rates or prevalence-type rates.

Consider the data in Table 4.11 that were obtained in the Collaborative Perinatal Project.[13] A weak association was noted between immunization with killed polio vaccine and stillbirth (RR = 21/18 = 1.2). However, it was observed that time of entry into the study was confounding: women who entered the study early had a higher exposure to killed polio vaccine and also had a higher rate of stillbirth. As seen in Table 4.12, the rate of stillbirth was 23/1000 in women who entered early and 17/1000 in those who entered late. The exposure to killed polio vaccine was 37% in the early group (5,464/14,955) and only 3.8% in the late group (1367/35,911).

To control for this confounding by time of entry, either direct or indirect standardization may be used. The formula for a directly standardized rate ratio is:

$$SRR = R'_1 \div R'_2 \qquad (4.4)$$

where R_1 is computed as in Formula 4.2. As illustrated in Table 4.12, the standardized rate of stillbirth in the exposed is 17.6/1000 and that for the nonexposed is 18.6/1000. The ratio of these two standardized rates is less than 1.0, indicating that the crude association between early exposure to killed polio vaccine and stillbirth was due to confounding by time of entry into the study.

Table 4.11
RELATION BETWEEN EXPOSURE TO KILLED POLIO VACCINE GIVEN DURING THE FIRST FOUR MONTHS OF PREGNANCY AND STILLBIRTH

| | Stillbirth | | | |
Exposure	Yes	No	Total	Rate
Yes	146	6,688	6,834	21/1000
No	799	43,264	44,063	18/1000
Total	945	49,952	50,897	

Table 4.12
RELATION BETWEEN EXPOSURE TO KILLED POLIO VACCINE GIVEN DURING THE FIRST FOUR MONTHS OF PREGNANCY AND STILLBIRTH, ACCORDING TO TIME OF ENTRY INTO STUDY

| Time of entry | Exposure | Stillbirth | | | Rate |
		Yes	No	Total	
Early[a]	Yes	125	5,339	5,464	23/1000
	No	213	9,278	9,491	22/1000
	Total	338	14,617	14,955	23/1000
Late	Yes	21	1,346	1,367	15/1000
	No	586	33,958	34,544	17/1000
	Total	607	35,304	35,911	17/1000

[a] Entry into study during first four months of pregnancy.

Directly Standardized Rate Ratio

$$SRR = \Sigma W_i\, r_{ij}/\Sigma W_i \div \Sigma W_i\, r_{ik}/\Sigma W_i$$

i = time stratum
j = exposure
k = no exposure

$R'_j = [14,955(125/5,464) + 35,911(21/1,367)] \div (14,955 + 35,911) = 17.6/1000$

$R'_k = [14,955(213/9,491) + 35,911(586/34,544)] \div (14,955 + 35,911) = 18.6/1000$

$SRR = R'_j/R'_k = 17.6/18.6 = 0.95$

Indirectly Standardized Rate Ratio

$$SRR = \Sigma a_i/\Sigma E(a_i) = (125 + 21) \div [5,464(213/9,491) + 1,367(586/34,544)] = 146/145.8 = 1.0$$

The weights used in the standardization were the total numbers of women who entered the study early and late. This is a common choice of weights. Another common choice is the numbers who entered early and late in the nonexposed group.[14] In the computation illustrated in Table 4.12, it can be seen that it is not necessary to compute the standardized rates, since division by the sum of the weights is done both in the numerator and the denominator. In essence, one computes the expected numbers of stillbirths in the standard population twice: once for the exposed group and once for the nonexposed group.

In this example, direct standardization posed no problem, since the stratum-specific rates were based on reasonably large numbers. However, suppose there were 12 strata rather than 2. In some of these strata the rate of stillbirth among the exposed might be based on small numbers. If there were one stratum with only one person among the exposed, the rate would be either 0/1000 or 1000/1000. Depending upon the size of the weight assigned to that stratum, (which would be determined by the size of the nonexposed group) the directly standardized rate might be very small or very large.

In such a situation, indirect standardization is preferable. The general formula for an indirectly-standardized rate ratio is:

$$SRR = \Sigma a_i / \Sigma E\ (a_i) \qquad\qquad (4.5)$$

where $E(a) = (a + b)c/(c + d)$. (Note that $E(a)$ in this formula differs from $E(a)$ in the computation of Chi-square.) As seen in Table 4.12, the indirectly-standardized rate ratio is 1.0, which differs only slightly from that obtained using direct standardization.

As indicated earlier, direct standardization is preferable if the stratum-specific rates are based on stable numbers. If two or more SRR are computed, they are also mutually comparable if the same weights are used. In computing an indirectly SRR, the weights used are those of the exposed group (see Table 4.12). Since these usually differ from one study group to another, two or more indirectly SRRs tend not to be comparable. However, indirect standardization is most useful in certain contexts, as will be illustrated in the section on standardized mortality ratios.

The stability of these SRR may be measured in the same manner as with crude rate ratios (Tables 4.1 and 4.2). Chi-square is a summary chi-square:[15]

$$X^2_1 = [\Sigma a_i - \Sigma E(a_i)]^2 / \Sigma V(a_i) \qquad\qquad (4.6)$$

where a_i, $E(a_i)$, and $V(a_i)$ are computed for each of the strata and summed. The 95% confidence interval is as in Table 4.1 and 4.2, with the substitution of the SRR for the rate ratio (RR). Note again that $E(a)$ in the Formula 4.6 is computed differently from $E(a)$ in Formula 4.5.

2. Standardized Odds Ratios

In most data from case-control studies, disease rates are not measured and the rate ratio must be approximated by the odds ratio. The standardized rate ratio is approximated by the Mantel-Haenszel odds ratio:[15]

$$\text{M-H OR} = \Sigma\ \frac{A_i D_i}{T_i} \div \Sigma\ \frac{B_i C_i}{T_i} \qquad\qquad (4.7)$$

Consider the data in Table 4.13, which were obtained in a study of children with cancer.[16] There was a crude association between prenatal X-ray and childhood cancer with an odds ratio of 2.1. However, birth order was associated both with X-ray expo-

Table 4.13

RELATION BETWEEN EXPOSURE TO PRENATAL X-RAY AND
CHILDHOOD CANCER, ACCORDING TO BIRTH ORDER

Birth order	Exposure	Childhood cancer Yes	No	M-H standardized odds ratio
First	Yes	85	36	$SOR = \dfrac{\Sigma A_i D_i}{T_i} \bigg/ \dfrac{\Sigma B_i C_i}{T_i} =$
	No	425	391	
	Total	510	427	$\left[\dfrac{(85)(391)}{937} + \dfrac{(93)(815)}{1661} \right] \div$
Other	Yes	93	57	
	No	696	815	$\left[\dfrac{(36)(425)}{937} + \dfrac{(57)(696)}{1661} \right] = 2.0$
	Total	789	872	

sure and with cancer and thus was confounding. Therefore, the data were stratified on birth order and a standardized odds ratio (SOR) was computed. The SOR was 2.0, indicating that the degree of confounding by birth order was minimal.

Computation of a SOR can readily be extended to three or more strata. For example, there could be four birth order strata (0, 1, 2, 3 +) or six birth order-sex strata (M − 0, 1, 2 + ; F − 0, 1, 2 +).

Computation of X^2 and the 95% confidence limits are as described under standardization of rates.

C. Standardized Mortality Ratios

A standardized mortality ratio (SMR) is a variant of an indirectly SRR. Since SMRs are in common use in occupational epidemiology, their derivation and use will be elaborated upon.

In the discussion of the analysis of incidence-type data, it was assumed that rates were available for both an exposed group and an unexposed group. However, frequently this is not the case. There may be an interest in comparing the mortality rate in some occupational group to the rate in the general population. For several reasons, general population rates may be considered preferable to rates in some "nonexposed group":

1.   They are readily available.
2.   They are based on large numbers and thus are stable.
3.   There may be no suitable nonexposed group.

Consider the data in Table 4.2. The crude rate ratio is the ratio between the rate in the exposed and the rate in the nonexposed. Suppose that the exposed group is all persons with a specific occupation. The nonexposed group, then, is all persons without that occupation. Obviously, in a general population the number of persons exposed is very small in relation to the number not exposed; the number not exposed differs only slightly from the number in the total population. If this population is followed for

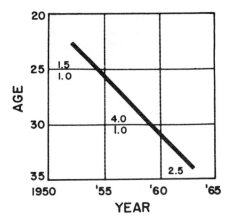

FIGURE 4.1.   Person-years experienced by
a person entering follow-up at age 23 in 1952
and leaving in 1962.

some period of time and incidence rates of disease measured, the rate in the total
population is a weighted average of the rates in the exposed and nonexposed groups.
However, since the exposed group is so small, the rate in the nonexposed group may
be approximated by the rate in the total population.

This approximation forms the basis of the SMR: population mortality rates are used
as a basis of comparison for the mortality rates in some group, be it occupational or
other. In this context "mortality ratio" is the ratio of the mortality rate in the exposed
occupational group to the rate in the total population. It is an approximation of a
crude rate ratio. "Standardized" means that potential confounding by some factor
has been controlled. Typically, in the computation of an SMR, age and time have been
controlled by indirect standardization. The formula for an SMR is:

$$SMR = 100 \times \Sigma a_i / \Sigma E(a_i) = 100 \times \text{Observed/Expected} \qquad (4.8)$$

where a_i is the number of persons with a specific cause of death in the ith stratum of
age and time and $E(a_i)$ is the number expected based on the age-time specific mortality
rates in the general population. By convention, 100 is multiplied times the observed/
expected ratio; in essence an SMR is the percentage of disease in the exposed as compared to the general population. Note that formulas 4.8 and 4.5 are essentially the
same. In the example of Table 4.2, for the ith stratum, $E(a) = PYRS_e (a + c)/PYRS_t$.

As indicated, age and time usually are controlled in an analysis using SMRs. Each
stratum consists of data similar to those in Table 4.2, specific for age and time. To
illustrate how these data are accumulated, consider Figure 4.1.[17] A person who enters
at age 23.5 on July 1, 1952, and who leaves on July 1, 1962, contributes 10 person-
years to the denominator of the study group. These are distributed as follows:

Time	Age	Person-years
1950—54	20—24	1.5
	25—29	1.0
1955—59	25—29	4.0
	30—34	1.0
1960—64	30—34	2.5
		10.0

Table 4.14
ILLUSTRATION OF COMPUTATION OF
STANDARDIZED MORTALITY RATIO (SMR)

Person-years

	Year		
Age	1950-54	1955-59	1960-64
20—24	1000	500	200
25—29	1000	1500	1000
30—34	500	500	1500

Observed deaths

20—24	2	1	0	
25—29	3	4	2	Σ Obs = 15
30—34	0	1	2	

Population rates (per 1000)

20—24	1.8	1.8	1.6
25—29	1.7	1.5	1.5
30—34	1.9	1.8	1.7

Expected deaths = population rates × person-years

20—24	1.8	0.9	0.3	
25—29	1.7	2.3	1.5	Σ Exp = 12.9
30—34	0.9	0.9	2.6	

SMR = 100 × Σ observed/Σ expected = 100 (15)/12.9 = 116

Of the nine potential strata illustrated in this table, this person contributes person-years to five.

Suppose that a number of persons contributed person-years to the example in Table 4.14. Each of the age-time-specific number of person-years is equivalent to the stratum specific PYRSe in Table 4.2. Each of the number of observed deaths is equivalent to the stratum specific "a" in Table 4.2. Each of the population rates is equivalent to the stratum-specific (a + c)/PYRSt in Table 4.2. Thus there are nine 2 × 2 tables illustrated in Table 4.14. For each stratum, the expected deaths E(a) is equal to the person-years times the population rate. The SMR is 100 times the observed/expected ratio. This is the same as indirect standardization.

In the usual computation of an SMR, age ranges from 20 to 100 or so and time may range from 1930 through 1975. Thus there are a large number of potential strata, with many of the strata having only a small number of deaths. Since the population rates are quite stable, indirect standardization is preferable to direct standardization.

Another feature of this computation lends itself to indirect standardization. In mortality studies, one usually is interested in evaluating observed and expected numbers of many individual causes of death. It is tedious to compute age-time specific rates for each cause in each study group. On the other hand the rates for the general population need only be computed once and then stored for retrieval. In order to compute the observed number of each cause of death, the data need only be read once to count the number dying from each cause. In the same reading of the data, the age-time-specific person-years can be computed for the study group. To compute the number expected for each cause, all that is needed is to multiply the matrix of person-years times the matrix of cause-specific death rates as illustrated in Table 4.14. This greatly reduces the time and cost needed for data analysis. A general computer program has been developed to use in SMR analyses.[17]

Analyses such as this are neither limited to occupational groups nor to mortality data. Any group with some experience can be the study group and morbidity rates rather than mortality rates may be used. For example, women with tuberculosis were followed to measure the incidence rate of breast cancer.[18] Expected number of breast cancers were computed on the basis of morbidity rates from the Connecticut Tumor Registry.

An SMR-type analysis may also be used in the direct comparison between two groups. If one wishes to compare disease rates between two study groups, computation of directly-standardized rates is preferable. An alternate method is to compute the expected number of cases of disease in one group on the basis of the rates in the second group. In the example of Table 4.2, $E(a) = PYRS_e(c/PYRS_o)$. In the example of Table 4.14, expected numbers would be computed for each of the strata and summed. This is the same as direct standardization with the weights being the age-time person-years distribution of the exposed group.

D. Proportional Mortality Ratios

A proportional mortality ratio (PMR) is another measure used frequently in occupational settings. In the computation of an SMR it is necessary to compute the person-years of follow-up of the study group. The number of person-years is needed for all persons in the study group. Frequently, however, the only information available comes from the death certificates of a group of persons with the same occupation (or with some other attribute). The basic data available are the cause of death, the age at death, and the date of death.

In a PMR, the expected number of deaths in a study group due to a specific cause are computed on the basis of the proportion (percentage) of that cause in the general population. As in an SMR, these expected numbers are age and time specific. (Strictly speaking a PMR should be called an SPMR or standardized proportional mortality ratio.) The total number expected is divided into the total number observed, as in an SMR:

$$\text{SPMR} = 100 \times \Sigma \text{ Observed}/\Sigma \text{ Expected} \qquad (4.9)$$

Consider the data in Table 4.1. Suppose that "a + b" is all deceased persons in a given occupational group. Then "a" is all persons dying of a given cause, say cancer. If, as in an SMR, "a + b" is small relative to "N", then the proportion of deceased persons in the general population who died from cancer is an approximation of the proportion in the nonexposed group. The expected value of "a" is therefore (a + b)(a + c)/N. An SPMR is computed as with an SMR, with observed and expected values being computed for each age-time stratum and summed.

The computation of an SPMR is illustrated in Table 4.15. The age-time distribution of all deaths in the study group is first presented. This is analogous to the person-years distribution in an SMR analysis. Next is the age-time distribution of death due to cancer in the study group. The population proportions of death due to cancer are analogous to the population death rates in the SMR computation. Finally, the expected deaths due to cancer are computed as in an SMR. In this example, death due to cancer occurs with twice the proportion expected based on the standard population.

Table 4.15
ILLUSTRATION OF COMPUTATION OF
PROPORTIONAL MORTALITY RATIO (PMR)

All deaths

	Year		
Age	1950—54	1955—59	1960—64
20—24	10	5	2
25—29	10	15	10
30—34	5	5	15

Observed deaths due to cancer

20—24	2	1	0	
25—29	3	4	2	Σ Obs = 15
30—34	0	1	2	

Population proportions of deaths due to cancer

20—24	0.07	0.07	0.07
25—29	0.09	0.10	0.10
30—34	0.11	0.12	0.12

Expected deaths due to cancer = population proportions × all deaths

20—24	0.7	0.4	0.1	
25—29	0.9	1.5	1.0	Σ Exp = 7.6
30—34	0.6	0.6	1.8	

SPMR = $100 \times \Sigma$ observed/Σ expected = 100 (15/7.6) = 197

For rare causes of death an SPMR is a reasonable approximation of an SMR which is a reasonable approximation of an SRR. As can be seen from comparing Tables 4.1 and 4.2, "a" and "a + c" are used both in computing SMRs and SPMRs. If, in general, the ratio (a + b):N is similar to the ratio $PYRS_e$:$PYRS_t$, the SPMR approximates the SMR. With uncommon causes of death this usually holds. However, when a cause of death is common (say 30% or more), the proportions a/(a + b) and (a + c)/N are large. This may mean that the disease under evaluation is common, or that relatively speaking all of the other causes of death are uncommon. While in general SPMRs are useful measures of association, they are less useful for common diseases such as cardiovascular disease.

The advantages of SPMR analyses are practical; much less time and money are needed to collect death certificates than to follow-up a number of persons. Also, the "healthy worker effect" is ignored in an SPMR analysis; by definition the ratio of observed to expected deaths for all causes is 1.0. Emperically, the interpretation of an SPMR is similar to the interpretation of an SMR.[19]

E. Matched Analyses

As indicated earlier, potential confounding may be controlled by matching in the design of a study. Matching is most often done in case-control studies. In a case-control study if there is concern that gender may be confounding, a male control can be matched to each male case and a female control can be matched to each female case.

In this situation, there is no association between gender and disease in the data since the proportion of males is the same in the cases as in the controls.

While my preference is to avoid matching in the selection of study subjects and to control confounding in the analysis, there are situations where matching may be preferred. There may be some factor that is known to be strongly associated with disease, so that if matching is not done, most of the cases will be persons with the factor (say males) and most of the controls will be persons without the factor (say females). If the factor is also related to exposure, extreme confounding will result that may not be amenable to control by stratification. In these situations there is no alternative to matching in the design.

Analysis of matched data should take into account that the study subjects were matched. Failure to do so may tend to lead to an error in the estimation of the rate ratio. However, if there turns out to be no association of the factor with the exposure, a matched analysis is not necessary.[20]

The general layout for the analysis of matched data is presented in Table 4.16.[21] The data are the same as in Table 4.7. In this study there was one case per control. The odds ratio is computed only on the basis of the discordant pairs: the number in which the case but not the control is exposed divided by the number in which the control but not the case is exposed.

It can be seen that the odds ratios computed from the matched data are essentially the same as those from the unmatched data. This means that within each sex, the factors upon which matching was done (age and neighborhood) were essentially not confounding. If it is necessary to control for other (unmatched) factors, the matching can be ignored.

More frequently, there are two or more controls per case. The data in Table 4.17 are the same as the data in Table 3.3.[22] The computation of odds ratio with more than one control per case has been presented.[23] In this example, the odds ratio from the matched analysis is 7.6. The odds ratio from the unmatched analysis is 7.1. It can be seen that in this example the two types of analysis gave similar results.

Many of the methods of analysis presented are routine and are based on repetitive operation. Because of the availability of the computer and of sophisticated calculators, general programs of analysis have been developed. In the analysis of data using SMR or proportional mortality ratios, a general program has been developed and is available.[17] Also, a number of analytic programs have been developed to use with a hand-held Hewlett-Packard 67 calculator.[27] The use of these general programs reduces the time needed to conduct epidemiologic analysis.

F. Multivariate Analysis

In assessing the possibility that an association between an exposure and a disease is due to confounding, the initial step is to determine which factors are associated with both exposure and disease. If only one factor is found to be so associated, control of confounding by stratification is straight-forward. If two or three factors are confounding, again, control by stratification is possible.

However, as the number of factors found to be associated both with exposure and disease increases, control by stratification becomes tedious. Also, the number of persons in each stratum becomes small and the SRR become subject to random variation. Multivariate techniques have been developed to control simultaneously for several confounding factors.[24-26] These techniques provide a useful adjunct to the simple, straight-forward stratification procedures of basic epidemiology.

Table 4.16
MATCHED DISPLAY OF DATA
RELATING EXPOSURE TO
COFFEE AND BLADDER CANCER

Men

Controls	Cases	
	Exposed	Not exposed
Exposed	4	43
Not exposed	69	364

$$RR \doteq OR = 69/43 = 1.60$$

Women

Controls	Cases	
	Exposed	Not exposed
Exposed	0	30
Not exposed	18	104

$$RR \doteq OR = 18/30 = 0.60$$

Table 4.17
HISTORY OF ESTROGEN USE AMONG
94 PATIENTS WITH ENDOMETRIAL
CANCER AND AMONG 188 MATCHED
CONTROLS

Case's use of estrogen	Control's use of estrogen			
	Both	One	None	Total
Yes	1	16	37	54
No	0	11	29	40
Total	1	27	66	94

$$RR \doteq OR = 7.6$$

V. COMMENT

In this chapter on analysis of data, common situations in epidemiology have been discussed. It is assumed that the amount of data available to analyze is reasonably large. Many of the formulas presented do not hold when the amount of data is small. Because of the basic inexactness in epidemiologic data and because epidemiology is nonexperimental, sophisticated analyses of small amounts of data are not likely to be productive. With small amounts of data either a given association is immediately obvious without analysis, as in the case of vinyl chloride and angiosarcoma, or it is not decipherable. Only by expanding the data available can understanding develop.

Many of the methods of analysis presented are routine and are based on repetitive operation. Because of the availability of the computer and of sophisticated calculators general programs of analysis have been developed. In the analysis of data using SMR or proportional mortality ratios, a general program has been developed and is available.[17] Also, a number of analytic programs have been developed to use with a handheld Hewlett-Packard 67 calculator.[27] The use of these general programs reduces the time needed to conduct epidemiologic analysis.

However, these and other programs must be used with caution. The data that are entered must be as accurate as possible and the results that are obtained must be subjected to careful scrutiny. An understanding of the bases of analysis is necessary to use such programs in a logical manner.

REFERENCES

1. MacMahon, B. and Pugh, T. F., *Epidemiology — Principles and Methods,* Little, Brown, Boston, 1970, 233.
2. Colton, T., *Statistics in Medicine,* Little, Brown, Boston, 1974, 174.
3. Arkin, H. and Colton, R. R., *Tables for Statisticians,* Barnes & Noble, New York, 1963.
4. Miettinen, O. S., Estimability and estimation in case-referent studies, *Am. J. Epidemiol.,* 103, 226, 1976.
5. Miettinen, O. S., Proportion of disease caused or prevented by a given exposure, trait or intervention, *Am. J. Epidemiol.,* 99, 325, 1974.
6. Cornfield, J. and Haenszel, W., Some aspects of retrospective studies, *J. Chronic Dis.,* 11, 523, 1960.
7. Cole, P. and MacMahon, B., Attributable risk percent in case-control studies, *Br. J. Prev. Soc. Med.,* 25, 242, 1971.
8. Nie, N. H., Hull, C. H., Jenkins, J. G., Steinbrenner, K., and Bent, D. H., *SPSS. Statistical Package for the Social Sciences,* McGraw-Hill, New York, 1970.
9. Monson, R. R., Rosenberg, L., Hartz, S. C., Shapiro, S., Heinonen, O. P., and Slone, D., Diphenylhydantoin and selected congenital malformations, *N. Engl. J. Med.,* 289, 1049, 1973.
10. Howe, G. R., Burch, J. D., Miller, A. B., Morrison, B., Gordon, P., Weldon, L., Chambers, L. W., Fodor, G., and Winsor, G. M., Artificial sweeteners and human bladder cancer, *Lancet,* 2, 578, 1977.
11. Colton, T., *Statistics in Medicine,* Little, Brown, Boston, 1974, chap. 2.
12. Armitage, P., *Statistical Methods in Medical Research,* Blackwell Scientific, Oxford, 1971, 387.
13. Slone, D., Heinonen, O. P., Monson, R. R., Shapiro, S., Hartz, S. C., and Rosenberg, L., Maternal drug exposure and fetal abnormalities, *Clin. Pharmacol. Ther.,* 14, 648, 1973.
14. Miettinen, O. S., Standardization of risk ratios, *Am. J. Epidemiol.,* 96, 383, 1973.
15. Mantel, N. and Haenszel, W., Statistical aspects of the analysis of data from retrospective studies of disease, *J. Nat. Cancer Inst.,* 22, 719, 1959.
16. Stewart, A., Webb, J., and Hewitt, D., A survey of childhood malignancies, *Br. Med. J.,* 1, 1495, 1958.
17. Monson, R. R., Analysis of relative survival and proportional mortality, *Comput. Biomed. Res.,* 7, 325, 1974.
18. Boice, J. D., Jr., and Monson, R. R., Breast cancer in women after repeated fluoroscopic examinations of the chest, *J. Nat. Cancer Inst.,* 59, 823, 1977.
19. Kupper, L. L., McMichael, A. J., Symons, M. J., and Most, B. M., On the utility of proportional mortality analyses, *J. Chronic Dis.,* 31, 15, 1978.
20. Miettinen, O. S., Matching and design efficiency in retrospective studies, *Am. J. Epidemiol.,* 91, 111, 1970.
21. Colton, T., *Statistics in Medicine,* Little, Brown, Boston, 1974, 171.
22. Ziel, H. K. and Finkle, W. D., Increased risk of endometrial cancer among users of conjugated estrogens, *N. Engl. J. Med.,* 293, 1167, 1975.
23. Miettinen, O. S., Estimation of relative risk from individually matched series, *Biometrics,* 26, 75, 1970.

24. **Miettinen, O. S.,** Stratification by a multivariate confounder score, *Am. J. Epidemiol.,* 104, 609, 1976.
25. **Holford, T. R., White, C., and Kelsey, J. L.,** Multivariate analysis for matched case-control studies, *Am. J. Epidemiol.,* 107, 245, 1978.
26. **Breslow, N. E., Day, N. E., Halvorsen, K. T., Prentice, R. L., Sabai, C.,** Estimation of multiple relative risk functions in matched case-control studies, *Am. J. Epidemiol.,* 108, 299, 1978.
27. **Rothman, K. R. and Boice, J. D., Jr.,** *Epidemiologic Analysis with a Programmable Calculator,* NIH Pub. No. 79-1649, Public Health Service, U.S. Department of Health, Education, and Welfare, Washington, D.C., 1979.

Chapter 5
THE INTERPRETATION OF EPIDEMIOLOGIC DATA

I. INTRODUCTION

The collection and analysis of epidemiologic data comprise the science of epidemiology. Knowledge of these methods is necessary in order to conduct epidemiologic research. Proficiency is gained primarily by practice.

The results of epidemiologic studies must be interpreted by epidemiologists and nonepidemiologists alike. In fact, in a given study the epidemiologist who has primary responsibility is perhaps among the least qualified to interpret the data. Interpretation of data is not limited to an inspection of the data collected, but includes an appraisal of the methods and of the primary epidemiologist.

Of equal importance is the necessity to view the results of any scientific study, epidemiologic or otherwise, in the context of other information. No one study is likely to provide a definitive answer to some question for all time. Today's facts may become tomorrow's fallacies. Therefore, the interpretation of all data must be viewed as tentative and subject to change. A modicum of caution must always be maintained.

Whereas opinions as to the meaning of any association seem in epidemiologic data will be varied, action to be taken based on the data must be definitive. Behavior will either be altered or it will stay the same. There is no room for equivocation. In the absence of a clear-cut interpretation of epidemiologic data, action must be prudent and err on the side of safety. There may be disagreement as to whether a substance in the workplace is a cause of cancer. Until more definitive data can be collected, the prudent action is to act as if the substance is in fact carcinogenic and reduce exposure to it.

Once it is recognized that the interpretation of data must be equivocal, and that actions to be taken must be prudent, the process of standard-setting can be seen to be political rather than scientific. Rarely will any data, epidemiologic or otherwise, be subject to unequivocal interpretation and resultant action. Even if there is agreement on the meaning of data in a given study, the extrapolation of the results to some other population is subject to controversy. The (potential) benefits to be gained by altering behavior must be judged in comparison to the (potential) costs.

In Chapters 2 to 4, the basic principles of epidemiologic research have been covered and the basic problems that may occur have been illustrated. Interpretation of epidemiologic data must take into account the possibility that any association between exposure and disease may be due to bias. The size of any association seen must be viewed in the context of the amount of data upon which the association is based as well as on the results of similar studies. It follows that persons who interpret epidemiologic data must be aware of the potential shortcomings of such data.

There are three steps in the process leading to the prevention of disease in humans. The first step is scientific: epidemiologists and other scientists design studies and collect data on the relationship between exposures and diseases. The third step is political: based on the judgments as to the meaning of epidemiologic and other scientific data, standards are set in the context of the potential benefits and costs. In between the scientific and political steps is one that is integrative and interpretive. Persons with knowledge of the scientific process must come to some agreement as to the meaning of current scientific data. Since these data usually derive not only from epidemiologic studies, the interpretation of data must take into account information from many

Table 5.1
A GUIDE TO STRENGTH OF
ASSOCIATION

Rate ratio		Strength of association
0.9—1.0	1.0—1.2	None
0.7—0.9	1.2—1.5	Weak
0.4—0.7	1.5—3.0	Moderate
0.1—0.4	3.0—10.0	Strong
<0.1	>10.0	Infinite

branches of science. In this chapter the scientific and integrative aspects of interpretation of epidemiologic data are considered.

II. THE RANGE OF RATE RATIOS

A primary purpose in epidemiology is to measure the association between exposure and disease. Information on each is collected and disease rates are computed in exposed and in nonexposed persons. The degree of association between exposure and disease is measured by a comparison of these rates.

The usual measure of exposure is the ratio between the rate of disease among the exposed and the rate of disease among the nonexposed: the rate ratio or the odds ratio. By definition, a rate ratio of 1.0 indicates no association; any other rate ratio indicates some association, either positive or negative. Since a rate ratio of exactly 1.0 is very unlikely, in most data an association between exposure and disease is present.

Practically speaking, however, ranges can be given to indicate the strength of association of a given rate ratio. As seen in Table 5.1, any rate ratio between 0.9 and 1.2 indicates essentially no association. This is not to say that the true association is in fact 1.0. It only means that associations in this range are too weak to be detected by epidemiologic methods. Note that this means if an exposure raises the rate of disease by 20% among the exposed, nonexperimental epidemiologic methods are unlikely to be able to detect this association. This has important bearing on the use of epidemiologic data in the setting of standards.

The ranges presented in Table 5.1 are totally empiric and based on experience. The cut-off points are clearly arbitrary and subject to redefinition. However, two general points are accepted by most epidemiologists:

1.   If the true association between exposure and disease is very weak, the detection of such an association by nonexperimental methods is unlikely.
2.   If the true association between exposure and disease is very strong, no epidemiologic expertise is necessary to detect it.

Two features of nonexperimental data from human populations are central to these general beliefs — variability and confounding. In situations where a true association is very weak, the range of variability in any data collected is large relative to the true rate ratio. That is, if the true rate ratio is 1.1, the observed rate ratio in five studies of the association may be 0.9, 1.0, 1.1, 1.2, and 1.3. Even with large numbers, simple random variation in a given study may lead to an observed rate ratio of 1.0. Likewise, if the true rate ratio is 1.0, in a given study an observed rate ratio of 1.2 would not be unexpected.

Confounding bias, also, is much more likely to influence the interpretation of small rate ratios than of large rate ratios. There may be one or more confounding factors that lead to a weak association between exposure and disease. An epidemiologist is limited in his ability to identify and measure such weak confounding factors.

At the other end of the scale, variability and confounding are much less likely to influence the interpretation of a large rate ratio. Even though in repeated studies a rate ratio may vary from 10 to 12 to 20, an association between exposure and diseases is clearly present. (The only caveat in such a situation is that the association be based on reasonably large numbers. As indicated in Chapter 4, if the number of exposed persons with disease is less than 5, any interpretation attached to the association must be extremely conservative). It is generally accepted that if some confounding factor exists that accounts totally for such a strong association, its detection should be relatively simple.

By contrast, the size of a rate ratio has little to do with the possibility that an association could be due to selection bias or observation bias. Either of these forms of bias can lead in data to a total misrepresentation of the underlying association between exposure and disease. Only through examination of the methods used in the selection of study participants and the collection of data can a judgement be made as to the likelihood of these forms of bias.

III. INTERPRETATION OF DATA WITH NO ASSOCIATION BETWEEN EXPOSURE AND DISEASE

A. Random Misclassification

Suppose that some exposure leads to some disease with a rate ratio of 5.0. If 100 exposed persons and 100 nonexposed persons are followed until the disease occurs, the data in the top third of Table 5.2 may result.

Suppose that some of the exposed persons were incorrectly classified as being nonexposed. The data in the middle third of Table 2 were the result. The rate ratio of 2.9 is less than the true rate ratio of 5.0, but still is greater than 1.0.

Suppose that there was no relation whatsoever between true exposure and classified exposure, so that a truly exposed person was equally likely to be called exposed or not exposed. The data in the bottom third of Table 2 might result. The rate ratio of 1.0 reflects the complete intermingling of exposed and nonexposed persons.

In a cohort study (or in an experiment) random misclassification results when there is imprecision in classifying someone as exposed or not exposed. The misclassification is random because it occurs with equal probability in diseased or nondiseased persons. In a case-control study, random misclassification results when there is imprecision in classifying someone as diseased or not diseased. The misclassification occurs with equal probability in exposed and nonexposed persons.

Random misclassification can only lead to a dampening of the rate ratio. A rate ratio greater than 1.0 is lessened while one less than 1.0 is raised. With complete random misclassification, the rate ratio is 1.0.

Consider the study of asbestos and lung cancer. Some of the persons in a cohort study said not to be exposed will in fact have had some asbestos exposure. The two groups are not "exposed and not exposed", but "heavily exposed and not so heavily exposed". Unless the random misclassification is extreme, a difference in exposure exists between the two groups. In the measurement of lung cancer in a case-control study, some persons called nondiseased will in fact have lung cancer. There simply would be an underestimation in the measure of the association between asbestos and lung cancer.

There may also an error in a cohort study in the classification of disease. If this

Table 5.2
EXAMPLE OF RANDOM
MISCLASSIFICATION IN A
COHORT STUDY

True measure of exposure

		Disease		
Exposure	Yes	No	Total	Rate
Yes	50	50	100	50/100
No	10	90	100	10/100

Rate ratio = 50/10 = 5.0

Partially misclassified exposure

Exposure	Yes	No	Total	Rate
Yes	40	40	80	50/100
No	20	100	120	17/100

Rate ratio = 50/17 = 2.9

Totally misclassified exposure

Exposure	Yes	No	Total	Rate
Yes	30	70	100	30/100
No	30	70	100	30/100

Rate ratio = 30/30 = 1.0

occurs equally among exposed and nonexposed groups, the rate ratio is not altered. (If this error has the potential to occur more in one group, observation bias will result.) In a case-control study, random error in the classification of exposure will not alter the ratio of exposure between case and control groups. However, in either type of study, the odds ratio will be dampened by this form of random misclassification.

Therefore, if an association between an exposure and a disease is found to be 1.0, random misclassification must be considered. If an association between an exposure and a disease is found to be other than 1.0, random misclassification could still have occurred. However, its effect would be only to tend to an underestimate of the true association.

B. Random Variation

All measures of association are subject to random variation. If some exposure is a cause of some disease with a rate ratio of 2.0, in some studies of the association a rate ratio of 1.0 may be found while in others the rate ratio may be 5.0. Any number can be substituted for each of the numbers in the preceeding sentence. The purpose of measures of stability (p-values or confidence intervals) is to quantitate the likelihood that associations of the size seen in a given study are due to random variation.

A basic assumption in the computation of measures of stability is that the rate ratio is unbiased. If doubts can be raised as to the validity of the size of the rate ratio, these doubts apply equally to the p-value and the confidence interval. It follows that the computation of a measure of stability for a crude rate ratio that has not been adjusted for any effects of confounding is of questionable value.

If the rate ratio seen in a study is 1.0, the size of the study is the major determinant of the measure of stability. If the study is large and if the rate of disease in the exposed (and nonexposed) is based on relatively large numbers of diseased persons, the confidence interval will be narrow, say 0.8 to 1.2. In such a situation, the likelihood that the true rate ratio is moderate or strong is quite low. However, if the study is small, the confidence interval may be wide, say 0.1 to 10.0. If the study were repeated, one would not be surprised to find a rate ratio of 5.0.

Thus, in a given study, a rate ratio of 1.0 should not be interpreted to mean that the exposure does not cause the disease. If the confidence interval is wide (if the study is based on only a few observations), repeated observations are needed. If in two or more studies, rate ratios of 1.0 are found, a more convincing case can be made that the exposure does not cause the disease.

C. Bias
1. Selection Bias; Observation Bias
Either of these forms of bias may lead to an observed rate ratio of 1.0 when the true rate ratio is other than 1.0. In order for such biases to mask any true nonunity rate ratio, the direction of the bias must be opposite to the direction of the true association between exposure and disease.

For example, suppose that drinking coffee leads to bladder cancer. If, in a case-control study, more complete coffee consumption histories are obtained from controls than from cases, the percentage of coffee drinkers in cases will be erroneously low, while the percentage in controls will be correct. This observation bias may counterbalance the true association and lead to an odds ratio of 1.0 in the study.

Such an example may be far-fetched, in that one would think an observation bias would in fact operate in the opposite direction. However, it does point out that in evaluating the likelihood of bias accounting for the results in a given study, the direction of the bias must be taken into account.

2. Confounding Bias
Confounding bias may lead to an observed rate ratio of 1.0 when the true rate ratio is other than one. As with the other forms of bias, the direction of the confounding must be opposite to the direction of the true association. This is "negative" confounding: some (confounding) cause of the disease is more common among the nonexposed than among the exposed.

In the analysis of data in which the crude rate ratio is 1.0, there is always a question as to how much pursuit of potential negative confounding is necessary. It may be argued that no association was seen because in the analysis "X" was not taken into account. While strictly speaking such a complaint is valid, the pursuit of potential negative confounding is usually futile. One can only assess the possibility of negative confounding for factors that have been measured. There always will be other potential negative confounders on which no data are available. Certainly, if important negative confounding is thought to exist, it should be evaluated. But the wholesale search for negative confounding is usually of little value.

IV. INTERPRETATION OF DATA WITH A POSITIVE ASSOCIATION BETWEEN EXPOSURE AND DISEASE

A. Bias
1. Selection Bias, Observation Bias
Either of these forms of bias may lead to an observed rate ratio different from the

true rate ratio. The crude rate ratio may be either less or more than the true rate ratio. The true rate ratio may have any value. Judgement as to whether selection bias or observation bias have led to a biased estimate of the true rate ratio is based totally on an evaluation of the design of the study and the methods of data collection.

Selection bias can be ruled out if the disease had not occurred when exposure was measured. Selection bias is unlikely in a case-control study if there was no knowledge of exposure when disease was diagnosed or in a retrospective cohort study if there was no knowledge of disease when exposure was measured. Selection bias should be considered especially when some exposure-disease association is postulated and when the authors appear eager to "prove" the association. The likelihood that persons with both exposure and disease were selectively enrolled into the study must be kept in mind.

Observation bias can never be ruled out. If disease was measured without knowledge of exposure, or if exposure was measured without knowledge of disease, observation bias is unlikely. However, since disease always follows exposure in time, absolute blindness in measurement of disease is not possible. At best, the methods used to measure disease in a cohort study or exposure in a case-control study must be absolutely comparable between the groups being compared.

Observation bias should be suspected when the specific association being evaluated is widely known to the participants in a study and to the persons conducting the study. Again, if the authors of a report appear to be eager to collect data to demonstrate the correctness of their prior notions, observation bias must be considered. The more neutral or disinterested an investigator appears to be, the less likely it should be that he has introduced bias into the collection of data.

2. Confounding Bias

As indicated in the chapter on analysis of data, the prevention or control of confounding bias is central to the conduct of epidemiological studies. Since it is difficult to demonstrate that negative confounding has led to a crude rate ratio of 1.0, the primary concern with confounding is that it has led to an erroneous appearance of association between an exposure and a disease that are unrelated.

In order to assess whether a given association is the result of confounding, it is necessary to know something about factors associated with the exposure or with the disease. In order for one or more of these factors to lead to confounding bias, it is necessary for the factor to be associated both with the exposure and the disease *in the study data.* If smoking is associated with coffee drinking in general, but if in a given study there is no association, smoking cannot be confounding in the association between coffee drinking and lung cancer.

The size of the crude rate ratio must also be considered in assessing the likelihood of confounding. For some factor to be a major source of confounding, its association with exposure and with disease must be at least as strong as the crude association between exposure and disease. Confounders with this characteristic are unusual or at least tend to be obvious when the crude association is moderate. However, a weak association ($RR < 1.5$) could readily be due in whole or in part to some confounding factor.

It is surprising how seldom confounding bias can be shown to account for some crude association between exposure and disease. While this undoubtedly reflects in part our imperfect knowledge of disease etiology, it also appears to be a fact of nature. Both negative and positive confounding factors are present in all populations, and there is some tendency for these factors to counterbalance each other. Confounding bias must always be considered as the reason for a given association; however, it must not be expected to be the reason for many associations.

B. Random Variation

As in situations where a rate ratio of 1.0 is observed, random variation is always a possible explanation for a rate ratio of any magnitude. Confidence limits give an indication of the range within which the true rate ratio is likely to lie, assuming that no bias is present. But no confidence interval, no matter how wide, is known to contain the true rate ratio, and no confidence interval, no matter how narrow, indicates that the true rate ratio is not 1.0.

In assessing the meaning of a rate ratio other than 1.0, the first and most important task is to judge the likelihood of bias. Since this is not only a quantitative process, the best guess as to the true rate ratio is not precise. Therefore, the upper and lower confidence limits are equally imprecise. The range between these limits is somewhat more precise as it largely reflects the size of the study. This range, rather than the size of the limits per se, best measures the stability of the rate ratio. A narrow range indicates a stable measure: a wide range indicates instability.

If a confidence interval does not contain 1.0, *and* if the ratio is judged to be free of bias, then a true rate ratio of 1.0 is unlikely. A real association between the exposure and the disease is a reasonable conclusion. The best measure of that association is the crude (or standardized) rate ratio. If data from more than one study are available and if the rate ratios in the several studies are similar, belief in a causal association is strengthened. This is true no matter what the size of the rate ratio. All that may vary is the strength of the association.

However, if the confidence interval contains 1.0, even though the rate ratio is judged to be free of bias, a true rate ratio of 1.0 is quite possible. The data in that study are simply too few to enable an unequivocal conclusion of association. This is true no matter what the size of the rate ratio. If data from more than one study are available and if the rate ratios in the several studies are similar, belief in a causal association is strengthened, even though each of the confidence intervals contains 1.0.

If a confidence interval contains 1.0, (or if the data are not "statistically significant"), this does not mean that there is no association between exposure and disease. It simply means that there are too few data upon which to base a firm conclusion of association. The best measure of the association is still the crude or standardized rate ratio. It is an error to conclude "no association" because a rate ratio does not differ from 1.0 at the 5% level of statistical significance.

C. Random Misclassification

As indicated earlier in this chapter, random misclassification tends to alter a rate ratio toward 1.0. Therefore, any rate ratio other than 1.0 cannot be simply a result of misclassification. If random misclassification has occurred, the true ratio must be more distant from 1.0 than the observed rate ratio.

This fact must be kept in mind in evaluating rate ratios other than 1.0. A study with a rate ratio of, say 2.0, cannot be excluded from consideration simply because disease or exposure were misclassified. At worst, the true rate ratio was underestimated. Such misclassification is likely in many studies where disease is not diagnosed by the best medical talent or technology. This does not necessarily invalidate the study.

V. INTERPRETATION OF DATA WITH A NEGATIVE ASSOCIATION BETWEEN EXPOSURE AND DISEASE

A causal association that is negative means that the exposure prevents or cures the disease. Interpretation of such an association is no different from interpretation of a positive association.

However, in searching for causes of disease, a negative association may be observed. While it is possible that working with some chemical prevents rather than causes cancer, there seems to be little evidence for such a postulate. More likely, a negative association between a chemical and a cancer is a result of chance or of bias.

In occupational settings, SMRs are frequently negative. This results because the mortality of a (healthy) worker population is being compared to the experience of a (healthy and unhealthy) general population. The negative association is a result of confounding by health status (the healthy worker effect).

For this reason, it is not inconceivable that an SMR less than 100 (rate ratio less than 1.0) could be seen for some disease that is in fact due to some condition of work. If the SMR for all cancer in 70 and the SMR for stomach cancer is 95, it is possible that the difference reflects some casual process. This must be kept in mind in evaluating occupational mortality studies.

VI. A SCHEME FOR INTERPRETATION OF DATA

A number of criteria have been suggested as steps to follow in the interpretation of data.[1-3] These criteria form a bridge between the interpretation of data from one study and the setting of standards based on the results of a number of studies. These criteria will be discussed in the context of occupational data.

A. Consistency

A consistent association is one that is seen in a variety of settings. In nonexperimental studies, especially, where biases are believed to arise from the nature, collection, and analysis of the data, an association seen in several studies is more believable than one seen only in one study.

A number of mortality studies have been conducted among workers in the rubber industry. In Table 5.3 are presented data from four different studies.[4] For none of the diseases is the SMR (100 × observed/expected) greater than 150. Each of these associations is weak. However, for stomach cancer and for leukemia, an excess is consistently seen in each study. This strengthens the belief that the association is causal.

For lung cancer and bladder cancer an excess is seen in some of the studies but not in others. This lack of consistency does not mean that some of the excesses are not causal. However, consistency cannot be invoked as an argument for causality. The presence of consistency argues for causality; its absence does not rule it out.

B. Specificity

In Table 5.3, the data are given for entire groups of rubber workers. Each group consists of persons who have worked in a variety of jobs and who have been exposed to a variety of materials. It is unlikely that each worker in each group shared any common pattern of exposure with any other worker. The excesses may reflect the combination of data from a small group of heavily exposed and diseased workers with data from a larger group of nonexposed and nondiseased workers.

In Table 5.4, the data on stomach cancer are given for persons who worked mainly with the raw materials used in rubber manufacture. The jobs of the persons in one study are not exactly the same as the jobs in another study, because of differences in classification of work areas. However, the excesses seen in these areas are relatively

Table 5.3
MORTALITY FROM SPECIFIC TYPES OF CANCER
AMONG FOUR GROUPS OF MALE RUBBER WORKERS

	Study I		Study II		Study III		Study IV	
Type of cancer[a]	Obs.	Exp.	Obs.	Exp.	Obs.	Exp.	Obs.	Exp.
Stomach	39	20.9	153	122.3	98	93.9	34	27.6
Lung	91	109.3	585	493.5	234	253.1	116	139.8
Bladder	9	12.3	60	38.9	48	39.5	21	18.1
Leukemia	16	12.5	28	23.3	55	43.0	25	18.1

[a] Slight differences exist in classification of type of cancer.

Table 5.4
OBSERVED AND EXPECTED NUMBERS
OF STOMACH CANCERS IN SELECTED
WORK AREAS[a]

Study	Work area	Observed	Expected
I	Compounding, mixing, milling	12	6.0
II	Tyres	65	48.0
III	Processing	18	9.9
IV	Compounding, mixing, milling	9	2.3

[a] Rubber is made in each of these areas.

much greater than those seen in the entire work force (Table 5.3). The association of stomach cancer and rubber making is relatively specific.

As with consistency, the lack of specificity does not mean that an association is not causal. There may be random misclassification because of the imprecise measure of exposure or of disease. There may be unrecognized harmful exposures present in dissimilar work areas. The presence of specificity argues for causality: its absence does not rule it out.

C. Strength of Association

As indicated earlier, epidemiologists generally believe that strong associations (high rate ratios) are unlikely to be due to unidentified confounding factors whereas weak associations could readily be due to confounding. However, the size of an association cannot be invoked as the only argument for causality. An SMR of 1000 (rate ratio of 10.0) may result from an observed/expected ratio of 3/0.3 or 30/3.0. Clearly, the second ratio is more suggestive of causality than the first. The size of an association must take into account the amount of data upon which it is based.

D. Dose-Response Relationships

Consider the data in Table 1.7, Chapter 1. The ranking of cigarette habit from non-smokers to former smokers to current smokers is a rough measure of lifetime dose of cigarette smoke. The rate of lung cancer of 10/100,000, 43/100,000, and 104/100,000 is an ordered response to the dose. The higher is the dose, the greater is the response.

As with high rate ratios, it is believed that confounding is an unlikely explanation for a dose-response relationship, and therefore a causal association is more likely.

While this does not necessarily hold, a rather complicated interrelationship must exist for a confounding factor to lead to the appearance of a dose-response relationship with a disease.

The lack of a dose-response relationship is fairly weak evidence against causality. The measure of exposure may be misclassified, there may be a threshold necessary for the exposure to cause the disease, there may be bias in the measure of exposure. The presence of a dose-response relationship is relatively strong evidence for causality.

E. Coherence

Coherence is essentially the same as believability. Included under coherence is the presence of some biologic mechanism to explain the association. Certainly the existence of a mechanism to explain the relationship between cause and effect is an important aspect of science. However, invoking a mechanism to assess the likelihood of causality is to put the cart before the horse. Judgment as to the interpretation of data from one or more studies should rely on the conduct of the studies and the data derived from the studies.

The issue of coherence is central to the setting of exposure standards. If a substance is found to be carcinogenic in animals, and if humans who are exposed to the substance have an excess of one or more cancers, one should certainly behave as if the substance is carcinogenic in humans. Even if a substance is known to be carcinogenic in animals, but no data suggesting carcinogenicity exist in human populations, prudence dictates limiting exposure to the substance. But it is improper to insist that because a substance is carcinogenic in animals, data must be found to show an excess of cancer in exposed persons before exposure is reduced. Such a procedure can only lead to a general lack of faith in epidemiologic data.

F. Temporal Relationship

A cause must precede an effect. An exposure must precede a disease if the exposure is to cause the disease. In most epidemiologic data, the decision as to whether exposure or disease occurred first can usually be inferred.

In cross-sectional studies, however, this is not the case. Exposure and disease are measured simultaneously. The possibility that exposure has been modified by the presence of disease must be kept in mind.

G. Statistical Significance

Throughout these pages caution is urged in the use of tests of statistical significance. A p-value or a confidence limit taken out of context has no meaning.[5] "Statistically significant" does not mean "associated", "causally associated," "meaningful" or "real." An association that is statistically significant is one that is based on sufficient data to exhibit some degree of stability. The measure of the association (rate ratio) may be totally in error. Certainly in repeated experimental studies, statistical significance bears a close relationship to the probability of random occurrence. But in individual nonexperimental studies, statistical significance must be interpreted with great caution.

REFERENCES

1. **Hill, A. B.,** *Principles of Medical Statistics,* Oxford University Press, New York, 1966, chap. XXIV.
2. **U.S. Department of Health, Education and Welfare,** *Smoking and Health,* PHS Publ. No. 1103, U.S. Government Printing Office, Washington, D.C., 1963, 182.
3. **Susser, M.,** *Causal Thinking in the Health Sciences,* Oxford University Press, New York, 1973, chap. 11.
4. **Monson, R. R.,** Effects of industrial environment on health, *Environ. Law,* 8, 663, 1978.
5. **Rothman, K. J.,** A show of confidence, *N. Engl. J. Med.,* 299, 1362, 1978.

Occupational Epidemiology

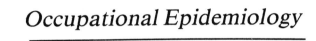

Chapter 6
STUDIES OF MORTALITY

I. INTRODUCTION

In assessing the possible effects of occupational exposures, an epidemiologic study may be designed to evaluate the general effects of an exposure or to measure the occurrence of a specific disease. In cohort studies more than one outcome is usually measured, even though there may be a specific interest in one disease. In case-control studies, one or several diseases usually are selected for investigation. In a cross sectional study, one or many diseases are evaluated in relation to one or many exposures. However, none of these general descriptions is hard and fast, and each of these methods can be used in the evaluation of occupational illnesses.

Mortality studies are typically retrospective cohort studies. A population of occupationally-exposed persons is assembled on the basis of past records and followed until the present to determine its mortality experience. Because of the necessity to determine the cause of death for each deceased member of the study cohort, it is logical to evaluate a number of causes of death. The observed numbers of death from each cause are counted and compared to the number expected, as computed by one or more methods.

The usual comparison population in a mortality study of an occupational group is some general population, frequently the entire U.S. population. Age-time-race-sex-cause specific rates are available in relatively great detail. These rates are multiplied times the age-time-race-sex specific person-years of follow-up of the study population in order to compute the number of deaths expected from each cause. One hundred times the ratio of observed to expected is the "standardized mortality ratio" (SMR).

Another means of computing the numbers of deaths expected from each cause is by the use of proportional mortality data. Rather than using mortality rates for the U.S. general population, expected numbers of specific causes of death are computed on the basis of the percentage of each cause out of the total number of deaths. Again in these computations age-time-race-sex specific computations are done.

The conduct of the "SMR" and "SPMR" studies in occupational settings is similar to the conduct of these studies in other settings. However, there are certain characteristics of data unique to occupational groups. Employed persons typically have a number of different work experiences throughout their lives that begin at different ages and times, last for different lengths of time, and are subject to a great variety of exposure to specific substances and conditions. Rather than simply having an exposure that is present or absent (yes or no), each person's work experience can be categorized in a variety of nonmutually exclusive ways. It is in the complexity of work histories that occupational mortality studies differ from other retrospective cohort studies.

On occasion it is more efficient to conduct a case-control study within a defined cohort of employed persons. All persons are followed to determine their vital status at the end of follow-up, but exposure histories are obtained only for persons who die of specified diseases and for selected controls. Such studies are performed when the cost of obtaining or reviewing old work histories is high or when the number in the cohort is large relative to the number of deceased persons. Such "case-control studies within a cohort" are used to minimize the cost in time and money of the study.

II. RETROSPECTIVE COHORT STUDIES (SMR STUDIES)

In this section the collection, analysis, and interpretation of data on mortality among an occupational group will be discussed. The procedures will be illustrated by examples from a mortality study of rubber workers.[1-4]

A. Study Rationale

Historically, most occupational disease has been thought of as an acute illness in response to current exposure to some toxic substance. Such illness develops as a relatively direct response to some substance in the work place; the exposure and the disease frequently overlap in time.

In recent years, concerns over the long-term effects of relatively low-level occupational exposures have increased. Central among these concerns is the question as to whether cancer may be caused by chemicals used in industry. The exposure to these chemicals is continuous over relatively long periods of time; the acute effects of such exposures are minimal; development of cancer or of other chronic diseases is insidious. The disease may not be diagnosed until after the individual has retired.

Retrospective cohort studies of mortality are the logical way to evaluate the possibility of long-term effects on health while working in industry. Any chronic disease that leads to death may be evaluated. Cancer specifically tends to be a fatal illness; its presence at death is usually indicated on the death certificate. Also, cancer is a fairly specific disease and is less subject to random misclassification than, say, one of the cardiovascular diseases. Therefore, the primary value of mortality studies in industry is to assess the association between cancer and occupational exposures. The evaluation of other fatal diseases can be carried out at the same time, but the utility of mortality studies of other diseases has thus far been of limited value.

It is obvious that in mortality studies the effects of the exposure of yesterday rather than the exposure of today are being evaluated. If some exposure causes some cancer, 10 to 30 years of continuous exposure may be necessary for cancer induction; an additional 10 to 20 years may be necessary for the cancer to be detected; an additional 10 to 20 years may pass before the person dies of the cancer. Thus it is not inconceivable that substances used in 1930 are responsible for cancer deaths in 1980.

It is equally obvious that if there is concern over the carcinogenicity in humans of some substance recently introduced in industry, a study of persons dying today will provide no information. It may not be until the year 2000 or later that any effect will be seen.

As with any study — epidemiologic or otherwise — mortality studies must be viewed in the context of other information. If exposures of today are similar to those of yesterday, mortality studies of past workers will provide useful information. Animal studies and in vitro tests must be used to supplement data from human populations. No one method may be used in all situations; a variety of methods must be used to evaluate a specific question.

B. Collection of Data on Mortality

1. Selection of Study Population

In a mortality study in an industrial setting, the potential study population is every person who ever worked in one or more plants. This includes persons who worked one day in 1944 and those who were hired yesterday. For reasons of cost, however, some truncation of the study population may be done. For example, persons who worked fewer than 2 or 5 or 10 years may not be included. On *a priori* grounds, it seems unlikely that short-term exposure will lead to some chronic disease. However, there is no guarantee that such is the case, and there is no scientific reason to truncate a study population. If funds are not a consideration or if the number of short-term workers is relatively small, all persons should be entered into the study. This includes persons currently employed.

Selection of the study population is usually done from the personnel records maintained by the company. On occasion, rosters of union members may be used to replace or supplement company records. As long as the records maintained on an active work force in the past are used, there is no danger of selection bias. These records are made out prior to death and reflect the experience of living persons only. However, if upon the retirement or death of a person, personnel records are altered or destroyed, selection bias may result. Obviously, if the personnel records of some fraction of deceased persons are destroyed, the mortality experience of the remainder will be far better than that of the study population.

I am not aware of selection bias having been introduced into an occupational mortality study because of the selective destruction of records of deceased persons. However, in two recent reports, selection bias is a possibility.

A group of workers in a New England plant became concerned about the effects on health of work. In particular, several of their co-workers died from cancer. To evaluate this question further, the workers collected death certificates for 86 of their deceased co-workers. While the process of collection is not known, it seems likely that the certificates for co-workers who had died from cancer were especially sought out. Of the 86 deceased persons, 25% had died from cancer whereas only 18% would have been expected on the basis of national rates (this was a proportional mortality evaluation). There appeared to be an excess of cancer. Subsequently, separate studies were done on the entire group of deceased persons independently by the company and by the National Institute for Occupational Safety and Health (NIOSH). The observed and expected percentages of cancer were the same (17%) in each study.[5,6] In initial evaluation there appeared to be an excess of cancer deaths because of probable selection bias. Definition of the study population did not rely simply on whether a deceased person had worked at the plant, but also may have included the fact that he had died from cancer. Clearly, such a selection procedure would lead to an excess of cancer among the deceased persons.

Selection bias is also a possible, but not known, explanation for an excess percentage of leukemia among a group of deceased employees in a nuclear shipyard.[7] A retired welder with leukemia was seen by a physician. The welder reported that several of his co-workers had died at an early age. This triggered a search for all deceased persons who had worked at the shipyard. By a search of death records in several New England States, 1772 deceased workers were identified. An attempt was made to interview the relatives of these employees to determine whether the employee had been exposed to radiation in his work at the shipyard. Out of 592 successful interviews 146 deceased workers were found to have been exposed to radiation. Of these 146, 6 had died from leukemia, whereas only about one would have been expected. While it is possible that there is a causal connection between radiation and leukemia among these workers, it is also possible that there was a selective search for radiation workers with leukemia. If the searchers asked living employees if they knew of anyone who had worked with radiation and who had died from leukemia, there would be a biased over-representation of these workers in the group of deceased persons.

Such selection bias may be avoided in two ways. First, only characteristics of exposure should be used to define the study population, even if everyone in the population is deceased. Second, if every person who ever worked at the plant is included in the study, no bias in selection is possible.

2. Information to be Collected

Information to be collected on individuals will be used for three basic purposes: follow-up, evaluation of the possible effects of the work environment, and evaluation of confounding. All of the information desired will not usually be available. Information that is available should be collected in some balance between what would be nice to have and what is practical. Frequently, an individual who has worked in one plant for a number of years has had a number of jobs. Frequently, the details of change from one job to another are still available from records. However, to abstract the finest detail on each worker is to make prohibitive the cost of the study.

Information needed for follow-up depends upon the type of follow-up to be conducted. If an intensive individual follow-up is to be conducted, information should include name, date of birth, social security number, name of spouse or other relative, last known address, and date last worked. If follow-up is to be carried out through the Social Security Administration, all that is needed is name and social security number.

Information needed for evaluation of possible effects of the work environment includes details of work history and the death certificate. It is in collecting the details of the work history that some balance is needed. A minimum is the date and age when employment in the plant started and the number of years worked in total. Also, it is important to know in which departments a person worked, when he started working in each department, and how long he worked in each department. If the work histories in a given plant are relatively simple, then the complete chronology of when a person entered each department and when he changed is useful. Frequently, however, changes were made yearly or more often, and the amount of data that might be collected is excessive. It must be kept in mind that epidemiology is an imprecise science and that the collection of complete, elaborate, precise work histories may be of marginal value.

Information needed for evaluation of confounding usually is not available. Such information includes previous and subsequent employment, personal habits such as smoking, drinking, and dietary histories, familial diseases, and other factors that are determinants of disease. While there is no question that having this information would be useful, it is not clear that the lack of such information is a major flaw. In order for a factor to be confounding, it must be associated both with exposure and disease. If a specific disease, say lung cancer, is associated with work in a specific department, in order for smoking to be a confounder, persons who work in that department must be heavier smokers than those who work elsewhere in that plant. While this is of course possible, it is not obvious that smokers preferentially take up specific forms of employment, especially within a specific plant.

Observation bias in the collection of information on exposure is unlikely provided that it is done without knowledge of information on outcome. Information on exposure was recorded prior to death and thus is unbiased. Only if this information is altered after death, or if it is collected in a different manner for deceased and living persons, can bias enter the data. On the other hand, random misclassification as to a person's exposure is always present. Even if a person's work history is available, this is only an approximation of the actual exposures. If an association between exposure and disease is found in spite of the inevitable random misclassification, the measure of the association can only be an underestimate.

Observation bias in the collection of information on disease is likely. In mortality studies such information is obtained solely from the death certificate. The basic comparison made is between cause-specific mortality in the study population and cause-specific mortality in the general population. The death certificates for the population are coded by experienced state nosologists. The death certificates for the study population usually are coded by the epidemiologist doing the study or by her designate. There is no guarantee of comparability of coding.

Comparability is a central concern in all epidemiology and is a specific concern in mortality studies. If the code assigned by the state nosologist is available, it should be used. Usually, however, this code is not written on the copy of the death certificate provided by the state, and it must be recoded. There is a temptation to code the disease as precisely as possible. To this end, autopsy or additional clinical information may be obtained so as to do a "better" job of disease coding. Such a procedure, however, introduces a gross lack of comparability between the study population and the general population. Whereas the death certificates for the study population may indeed be more accurate, the important issue is comparability. In order for a comparison to be made between the general population and the study population, the death certificates must have been coded in the same manner.

The issue of coding of death certificates is of importance only if published mortality rates for a general population are to be used in comparison with the rates of a study population. If internal comparisons within the study population are to be made, for example, between the employees of two departments, any coding scheme for the death certificates may be used as long as the scheme is the same for the members of each department.

3. Follow-Up

Three basic sources are used in the follow-up of employee populations: company records, the Social Security Administration, and others.

Company records are used to determine the number of persons who are still actually employed and to identify those who died either while employed or while covered by a death benefit plan. They provide relatively complete information for these workers. Also, if there is active contact with retirees, living retirees can be identified.

Social Security records are used to identify persons in the study population for whom a death claim has been filed. The Social Security number and the final six letters of the last name are provided to the Social Security Administration (SSA). In return, the SSA gives for each person known to be deceased the date of the death claim and the state of death or the state from which the claim was filed. In addition, a frequency distribution is given for the number of persons currently paying into the system, those for whom claims have been filed or are being paid, and those on whom no information is available. There is no guarantee that all deceased persons are identified through the SSA, for if a person dies but no death claim is filed, the SSA will not know of the death. The magnitude of the error introduced by the lack of death claims is difficult to estimate, but it probably is not large.

A large variety of other sources of follow-up have been used.[8,9] With sufficient time and money, at least 90% follow-up is possible. While a high degree of follow-up is desirable, a relatively low percentage does not necessarily invalidate a study. This will be discussed further in this chapter under analysis of data.

Death certificates are obtained either through company resources or through state health departments. As indicated above, the best code for the cause of death is that assigned by the state. If that is lacking, the certificates should be coded by a trained nosologist who codes in a manner similar to that done by governmental nosologists. There must be comparability between the codes used for the general population and the study population.

Another problem in the coding of death certificates is in the International Classification of Diseases (ICD).[10] Every 10 years or so, there is a change in the numbering system used to code diseases and cause of death. Because changes in the understanding of the processes of disease and because of changes in medical fashions, diseases and their interrelationships change. For example, before 1949 leukemia was coded as a disease of the blood; since that time it is grouped with the malignant neoplasms. Also, the rules of filling out and coding death certificates change from time to time.

In the analysis of causes of death, all deaths should be coded according to the same ICD revision. Therefore, certificates must be recoded from one ICD revision to another. It is inevitable that in such recoding some inaccuracy is introduced. While there are fairly precise rules as to comparability from one ICD revision to the next, the coding still must be recognized as a procedure carried out by humans. Death certificates are filled out by physicians who have an imperfect understanding of the process which led to death. Usually autopsy information is not on the death certificate. Death certificates are coded by nosologists who are well trained in their craft. However, there is no question that from place to place and from time to time there are nonmeasurable differences in the filling out and coding of death certificates.

In spite of the variability inherent in the use of death certificates, the basic test lies in how useful they have proved to be in practice. Rates based on these certificates are relatively stable from time to time and from place to place. In general there are no major changes in rates for specific diseases from one ICD revision to the next. For diseases such as cancer, the regularity of mortality rates reflects the basic recognition of John Graunt that data on human populations are remarkably stable. For cardiovascular diseases, however, where clinical and pathological knowledge change from era to era, mortality rates of specific conditions reflect these changes.

Sufficient experience has been accumulated with death certificates and published mortality rates to prove their utility. Certainly caution must continue to be maintained in the use of such data. But there is no question that mortality studies on industrial populations have been and will be an important source of data on human health and disease.

C. Analysis of Data on Mortality
1. Data Points to be Defined for Individuals and Apportionment of Person-Years

Figure 4.1 presents the basic compilation of person-years for an individual and how those person-years are apportioned by age and calendar time. In Figure 6.1, specific important points in a person's work experience are also considered.

In occupational mortality studies, follow-up for an individual may not start when the individual is first employed. Whereas it may be possible to define a cohort on the basis of records dating back to 1900, there may be no feasible way of identifying persons who have died until 1940. In particular, since the Social Security Administration was not founded until 1937, no follow-up through its records is possible before that time. The solution is not to eliminate persons who started working before the start of follow-up, but to count their person-years only since the start of followup. For the person illustrated in Figure 6.1, follow-up starts at age 40 in 1940 and continues for 40 years.

Once follow-up begins, it must continue until death, until the end of the study (live withdrawal), or until the person is lost-to-follow-up. If the person in Figure 6.1 had been laid off between 1945 and 1950, his follow-up would have continued. Once a person is lost, he may not reenter. However, note that the start of follow-up can be moved forward in time. If it is desired to follow only persons who worked in department "Z", this individual would not enter follow-up until 1950.

Expected numbers of specific causes of death are computed for each individual by multiplying his age-time specific person-years by the age-time-cause specific rates of death for persons of his sex and race. These expected numbers are invariate for each person, and are usually distributed into 5-year age-time groups.

In describing the mortality experience of a group of employed persons, several descriptive patterns may be used. The first is based on age and year of starting work. All persons who started work between ages 20 and 24 and in 1920-24 are grouped

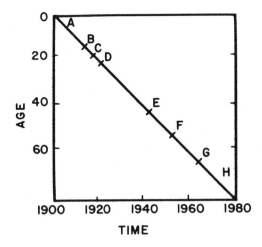

FIGURE 6.1.   Important points in a person's work experience.

Points	Lines
A. Born 1/1/1900	(C-B) = Years worked in dept. X
B. Started work, age 18, department X	(D-C) = Years laid off
C. Laid off, age 20	(G-B)—(D-C) = Total years worked
D. Rehired, age 22, department Y	(H-E) = Years followed
E. Follow-up started, age 40	(H-B) = "Latency," following initial
F. Transferred to department Z, age 50	employment in department X
G. Retired, age 65	(H-D) = "Latency" following initial
H. Died, 12/30/79, age 79	employment in department Y

together and their person-years and expected and observed numbers of deaths computed. The person illustrated in Figure 6.1 would contribute 40 person-years to the 1920—24, age 20 to 24 cell. These person-years are independent of those for persons who started work between ages 25 and 29 in 1920—24, etc. By inspection of the observed/expected pattern of mortality according to age and time started working, an impression is gained as to whether any excess is observed among persons who started work at a certain time period or age. In this example, when a person dies, he is categorized under his age and year of employment.

A second common descriptive pattern is age and year of death. Person-years are distributed for each age and time period in which an individual is followed. The person illustrated in Figure 6.1 would contribute 5 person-years to the 1940—44, age 40 to 44 cell and 5 person-years to seven other cells for a total of 40 person-years. His death would be categorized in the 1975-79, age 75-79 cell. By inspection of this pattern of observed and expected numbers, an impression is gained as to the era and ages in which any excess has been seen.

A third descriptive pattern is years worked by latency. Years worked may either be total years in a plant or only the number of years in a given department. If years worked in a department are used, follow-up does not start until the person entered the department of interest, since he could not have died prior to having entered that specific department.   Latency is somewhat of a misnomer, since it suggests the length of time a disease was present but not manifest. The definition of latency in the follow-up context is the total length of time between start of work and end of follow-up. However, it is difficult to separate "latency" into its three logical component parts: years of exposure needed to induce disease, years needed for induced disease to become

Table 6.1
OBSERVED AND EXPECTED[a] DEATHS AMONG A
COHORT OF 13,571 RUBBER WORKERS[b]

ICD no.[c]	Cause of death	Observed deaths	Expected deaths	SMR[d]
—	All causes	5079	6090.6	83
140—205	All cancers	986	1064.9	93
150—159	Digestive	368	364.1	101
151	Stomach	98	90.4	108
153	Large intestine	104	103.4	101
160—164	Respiratory	255	293.4	87
177—181	Genitourinary	155	159.6	97
181	Bladder	48	39.5	122
200—205	Lymphatic and he-matopoietic	105	94.4	111
204	Leukemia	55	42.7	129
330—334	Vascular diseases of central nervous system	493	524.0	94
400—468	Circulatory diseases	2448	2871.8	85
470—527	Respiratory diseases	218	327.0	67
530—587	Digestive diseases	217	279.0	78
590—637	Genitourinary diseases	75	135.8	55
800—999	Accidents, poisoning, violence	279	440.1	63
—	Residual	363	448.0	81

[a] Expected deaths computed on basis of age-time-cause specific mortality rates for U.S. white males.

[b] Observed and expected numbers differ slightly from those previously published; some death certificates were recoded; expected deaths were re-computed using updated death rates.

[c] International Classification of Disease, 7th Revision.

[d] Standardized Mortality Ratio = 100 × observed/expected.

manifest, and years between disease manifestation and death. At a minimum, no one of these periods can be longer than the number of years defined as "latency".

Care must be taken in apportioning person-years according to years worked and latency. One does not simply stratify a population into those who worked specific number of years and follow each group independently. Persons who worked 10 years contribute 5 person-years to the 0 to 4 stratum and 5 person-years to the 5 to 9 stratum. All 10 person-years should not be placed in the 5 to 9 stratum. An example of this problem has been discussed.[11,12] Also, the number of years a person has worked must be equal to or less than "latency".

The person illustrated in Figure 6.1 worked for 45 years. His latency was 62 years. However, he was followed for only 40 years. In an analysis of person-years (and expected numbers) by years worked by latency, he would enter in the (20 to 24, 20 to 24) cell. He was not under active follow-up for the first 20 years of years worked or of latency. He would contribute 5 person-years to each years worked stratum through that of the (40 to 44) stratum, and 15 person-years to the (45 to 49) stratum.

2. Dealing with Persons Lost-To-Follow-Up

It is desirable to determine the vital status at of the end of the potential period of follow-up for all persons. Usually, however, this is not possible. There always are some persons who are not traceable. Such persons must be considered to be under follow-up only for the known period of observation, say the years during which they worked. Note that if some mass form of follow-up is used, such as the SSA, it may not be known which persons not known to be dead are still alive and which are lost. In this event, all nondead persons usually are considered to be alive at the end of follow-up.

If an individual follow-up has been carried out, four basic assumptions can be made about persons who are lost-to-follow-up:[13]

1. They may be eliminated from the study.
2. They may be assumed to be deceased at the end of follow-up.
3. They may be assumed to be alive at the end of follow-up.
4. They may be assumed to be lost at the date of loss.

Assumption one is usually not advisable. All persons once they are entered into follow-up are at risk of dying and contribute to the number of deaths expected in the study cohort. If they are excluded, the expected numbers of deaths will be artificially low. However, if the observed deaths are fewer than the expected, even with the exclusion of the lost persons, any error introduced leads to a conservative interpretation of the data. The cohort only appears to be less healthy than it actually is.

Assumption two is usually not realistic. It usually is easier to identify deceased persons than living persons, since death certificates and insurance claims are made out at time of death. It is unlikely that a person would become lost simply because he dies. However, if the observed deaths are fewer than those expected even with this extreme assumption, a conservative interpretation of the data again results.

Assumption three is the most conservative assumption if an excess of some cause of death is seen. In this event, all of the observed deaths due to that cause probably have not been identified, and the number of deaths expected is maximal. If even with these two opposing errors in measurement an excess is seen, it is an underestimate of the true excess. However, if no excesses of specific causes are seen using assumption three, then a reanalysis should be made using assumption four.

Assumption four is probably the most realistic assumption in most studies. It assumes that the mortality of persons who were lost does not differ from the mortality of persons who continued under follow-up. While this is clearly a guess, I am not aware of any data that would suggest that in general this is not the case. Assumption four and assumption three provide reasonable lower limits and upper limits as to the range of the numbers of deaths expected from the various causes.

In presenting data as to percentage of follow-up, the usual method is to give the percentage of persons who were followed until death or until the end of the study. This method tends to be unnecessarily conservative. Most persons who become lost to follow-up are followed for some number of years and contribute to the person-years and the expected numbers of death. Instead of computing the percentage of persons followed, one could compute the percentage of the maximum number of person-years or the percentage of the maximum number of expected deaths from all causes. Either of these percentages will usually be greater than the percentages of persons followed. For example, in a study of rubber workers only 69% of white male union members were followed until death or end-of-follow-up through company records.[1] However, the follow-up through these records represented 75% of the potential maximum person-years of follow-up and 82% of the maximum number of expected deaths from all causes. In describing follow-up data, all three of these percentages could be presented.

3. External vs. Internal Comparisons

In an external comparison the mortality in the study population is compared to the mortality in some general population. Usually the number of deaths from specific causes observed in the study population is compared to the number expected based on the mortality rates in the general population (see Chapter 4). One hundred times the observed/expected ratio is the "standardized mortality ratio" or SMR. These computations are an example of indirect standardization.

The computation of SMRs has been used in occupational studies for many years. Among the reasons for the continued use of SMRs are:

1.   The general population rates are based on large numbers and are stable.
2.   There may be no better comparison population to serve as a control group for the employed population of interest.
3.   Time and money are saved by using previously assembled population rates.
4.   Results of SMR studies are in general believable.

If only one group is compared to the general population, there is little disagreement over the use of SMRs. However, if the mortality experiences of two or more groups are to be compared to a general population, objections may be raised to the use of SMRs. Since an SMR uses indirect standardization, the weights used as standards derive from each study group rather than from the outside population. Even though an SMR is age-standardized, sets of SMRs are not necessarily mutually comparable, since the age distributions of the study groups may differ.

This potential problem with indirect standardization is simply one of potential confounding by age. If the age distributions of two or more study groups differ, *and* if the SMR differs from one age to another, the SMRs from the individual groups are not comparable even though each by itself is comparable to the outside population from which the standard rates derive.

Note that if either the age distributions of the individual study groups are the same (or differ little), *or* if the SMR is (relatively) constant from one age group to the next, two overall SMRs can be compared directly just as can two directly standardized rate ratios. Further, if one group is appreciably older than a second, if the SMR is higher at older ages, and if the older group has a higher SMR than the younger, the difference in SMRs is real. The *reason* for the higher SMR in the older group is not that this group has been exposed to a more dangerous environment, but rather that they are older. Whether the younger group will experience higher SMRs at older ages remains to be seen.

In an internal comparison the mortality rates for one cause of death are compared among two or more study groups. Usually, the rates in each group are directly compared using direct standardization. The age-specific rates in each group are weighted by some common age distribution. The resultant standardized rates are directly comparable. This comparability is a definite advantage for direct standardization.

The primary disadvantage of direct standardization is in the basic instability of the stratum-specific rates derived for each study group. While this can be overcome to some extent by combination of data cells or strata, the process of direct standardization tends to be costly and tedious. Another disadvantage is that if one group has a rate higher than a second group, it is unknown whether the first is too high or the second is abnormally low.

Because of the efficiency of indirect standardization and because of its demonstrated utility, I rely on the computation of SMRs for screening large amounts of data and for all preliminary analyses. Also, even when evaluating the mortality experience of two or more groups, I rely exclusively on SMRs when there is no specific reason to compare each group to the other.

If after the computation of SMR, excesses are seen, and if there is a desire to compare two or more groups directly, and if the age distributions of these groups differ, than direct standardization is indicated. The most common situation where direct standardization would be useful is where there are two or more levels of exposure to some hazardous substance and where a dose-response relationship between exposure and disease is being evaluated.

There are situations in occupational data where even direct standardization does not guarantee age (or age-time) comparability. If one is evaluating mortality patterns by age and calendar time, one age group obviously has an age distribution different from other age groups. If one is evaluating mortality patterns by age and year started working, there is a correlation between chronological age and age started working; there is a question as to who is to be compared to whom. One can compare the mortality rates of persons at similar chronological ages or of similar ages started working. However, it is not possible to control each simultaneously. If one group started in 1955 at age 25 and a second in 1955 at age 35, either the two groups differ by 10 years in age (at the same calendar time) or by 10 years in time (at the same age). Finally, if one is evaluating mortality patterns by years worked and latency, it is not possible to control simultaneously for age, time, age started working, and time started working.

4. The Healthy Worker Effect

The healthy worker effect (HWE) is a name given to the observation that employed populations tend to have a lower mortality experience than does the general population.[14,15] This is not surprising, since at least initially, persons entering the work force would be expected to be drawn from the healthier segment of the general population. Persons with life-shortening disease tend to be less likely to become employed; the mortality rate of a general population is a weighted average of rates of the healthy and the unhealthy.

As an employed population ages, the HWE decreases, that is, the SMR becomes closer to 100.[14] This does not necessarily mean that the employed population is becoming less healthy. It may only be the natural result of the increasing mortality with age. If there is some absolute reduction in an employed population's mortality rate at all ages, this will become relatively less with time as the population gets older. The baseline rate of death will increase as the population ages and the reduction due to the "healthiness" of the population will become an increasingly smaller percentage of the overall rate.

The HWE tends to be stronger for nonmalignant diseases than for cancer.[14,15] This makes intuitive sense, for cancer tends to occur at older ages. Of the persons who eventually die from cancer, few have manifest disease in the 20s when most persons begin employment. However, of persons who eventually die of diabetes, or of asthma, or of rheumatic heart disease, many would have the disease at age 20 and may be less likely to enter the work force.

5. Active vs. Retired Employees

In analyzing data on employed groups, there may be a desire to compare the mortality experience of active persons with that of retired persons. Such a comparison may lead to a difficulty in interpretation. Persons who retire before age 65 frequently do so for health reasons. It would be expected that their mortality experience would be poorer than that of persons who continue working. This would be the case whether or not a person's poor health was due to occupational exposures. It is more logical to stratify on age, say less than 65 vs. 65 and above.

D. Interpretation of Data on Mortality

As indicated in Chapter 5, the strongest evidence that an association is causal derives from situations where the same association is seen in two or more independent groups. Because of the nonexperimental source of data on humans and because of the nonmeasurable biases likely to affect the data, it is unusual for one data source to allow unequivocal conclusions about an occupational exposure and a disease.

In assessing mortality data, one usually is considering an observed number, an expected number, and an SMR. If the expected number is very small, say less than two, the SMR must be very large, say 1000 or greater, in order for one to consider seriously the possibility of a causal association. As the expected number increases, a lower SMR than 1000 becomes of concern as reflecting a causal association. However, even with large expected numbers, an SMR of 150 or less is difficult to interpret. In such a situation, the possibility must be considered that there is some subgroup in the population with a high SMR counterbalanced by a larger subgroup with an SMR of 100 or less.

Because of the HWE, however, even SMRs less than 100 may be of concern. If the all causes SMR is 70 and the all cancer SMR is 95, one should consider the possibility that some persons developed cancer because of their work. While this must not necessarily be so, neither is it necessary that an SMR of 95 for all cancer means that no cancer resulted from the work.

E. Example — Rubber Workers

In 1971 the six major U.S. rubber companies together with the United Rubber, Cork, Linoleum, and Plastic Workers of America contracted with the Harvard School of Public Health and with the University of North Carolina School of Public Health to study the health of rubber workers. A study of the mortality experience of B. F. Goodrich employees in Akron, Ohio was conducted.[1-4] Four groups were defined: white male union members, white male salaried employees, all black males, and all females. In this example only the 13,571 white male union members who were employed on or after January 1, 1940, will be discussed.

1. Data Collection

For each person who ever worked at this plant, the Company maintained a file card containing name, race, social security number, date of birth, service date, date last employed, and last department of employment (service date was the date first employed, adjusted for lay-offs). While this amount of information was sufficient to conduct a follow-up study, the small amount of information on work history limited the potential value of the study.

The maximum amount of potential information on an employee's work history was contained in the personnel folder. In these folders a complete record was kept of a person's work experience, including department of employment and jobs worked and the amount of job changes; tens and even hundreds of different department-job descriptions were available. The abstraction of this volume of data would have been expensive.

Because of a policy instituted during the 1960s, personnel folders were destroyed 10 years after an employee left work. Therefore, for the majority of former employees, no personnel record was available. However, Local #5 of the United Rubber Workers had maintained dues file cards for each union member since 1933. On these cards was entered in sequence the department in which an employee worked. From these cards it was possible to determine in which departments an employee had worked and the approximate number of years spent in each department. The only other useful information on the card was name and social security number. Since this information was also on the Company file card, data from the two sources could be merged.

No selection bias was possible in the definition of the study population, since the records were filled out prior to death. None of these records was destroyed and all of these records were abstracted.

Since the information on the file card maintained by the Company was straightforward and simple to find, abstraction was done directly with a typewriter. Clerks typed the desired information onto a sheet of paper that could be read directly by a machine (Optical Character Recognition). Were this information being abstracted today, a teletype terminal or cathode ray tube terminal could be used and the data could go directly onto a computer disk. A program could be written to check for logical or range errors at the time of entry, so that insofar as possible, no erroneous data would be recorded.

By contrast, the departmental information contained on the Union records was relatively difficult to abstract. It was necessary to look through a number of cards to determine the order in which the department numbers had been entered and the years when a person changed jobs. To abstract each record 5 to 10 min were required. Therefore the information was entered onto Optical Scan forms by marking numbered boxes. These forms were then read by machine. Were this information being collected today, the same procedure would be used.

The abstraction of these two types of records illustrates different modes of data abstraction. If the data to be abstracted are readily recognizable and easy to abstract, a rapid, repetitive abstraction system can be developed. Essentially no thinking is needed to abstract the information, and the abstraction procedure can be geared toward speed without sacrificing accuracy. However, if the data are complex and require searching and thinking, the abstraction procedure must reflect this need. Rather than aiming at rapid abstraction, accuracy must be emphasized. The form should reflect the tasks of the persons who will use it.

The general principle to be followed in abstracting data from records is that the same person should not have to think carefully or search thoroughly and then enter the data rapidly and automatically. Also, some persons are more suited to careful and slow searching, and others are more suited to rapid abstracting. The person should be matched to the type of procedure to be used.

No observation bias was possible at this stage of data collection, since no information on outcome (cause of death) was available.

Approximately 32,000 white male union members were identified as having worked at this plant between the early 1900s and 1971. Over 18,000 of these men had worked for fewer than 5 years. For reasons of economy, only the 13,571 men who had worked five or more years were included in the follow-up.

Follow-up was carried out using company records, Internal Revenue Service records, and Social Security Administration records. Some persons were still actively employed; others were known to be retired. The two groups were known to be alive as of the date of abstraction.

A number of persons were determined to be deceased using Company records. These were men who had died while actively employed or while on vested rights status, that is, workers who had worked sufficient years (usually ten or more) to be eligible for death benefits.

The identification of the above groups of living and deceased persons was straightforward. However, there were over 4000 men who had worked for at least 5 years, who had terminated without vested rights, and who were not known to be dead. The tracing of these "terminated" employees is always difficult and time-consuming.

While in data analysis certain assumptions can be made, it is always preferable to determine the current vital status of each of these persons.

In the study being described, the 4000 + names coupled with social security numbers were first sent to the Internal Revenue Service (IRS). The IRS provided information as to whether an income tax return had been filed in a recent year. If a claim had been filed, the person presumably was alive as of that date. The IRS no longer provides this service.

Names and social security numbers of persons not located through the IRS were next sent to the Social Security Administration (SSA). Of the 1515 names submitted to the SSA, 739 were reported to be deceased.

Of the 13,571 men in the study cohort who had worked at B. F. Goodrich between 1940 and 1971, 4340 were determined to be deceased from company records and 739 were identified as being deceased through the SSA. Death certificates were obtained either from the Company or from the individual state health departments. The certificates were coded by a nosologist familiar with the coding procedures in effect at the time of death and then were recorded to the 7th International Classification of Diseases (ICD) for analysis. This was necessary so that there was consistency in the data to be analyzed.

Both selection bias and observation bias were possible at this phase of data collection. From company records a number of persons who were not in the study cohort were identified as being deceased. Inclusion of these workers would have led to selection bias, since they would have been included because they were deceased, not simply because they were rubber workers. By not including them, the study was smaller and less efficient, but was not biased.

Observation bias is always present in dealing with death certificates. Even if the ICD code from the states is available, it may not be the same as that assigned in Washington and coded for published vital statistics. Also, if recoding from one revision to another is done, this is subject to error and differences of opinion. If mortality rates are being compared within a cohort, and not externally, these errors tend only to random misclassiciation as long as they are independent of exposure group.

The observation bias in death certificates tends to differ by cause of death. For individual cancers, little bias is likely since the disease process and words used to describe the process are straightforward. However, for cardiovascular diseases and the nonmalignant diseases of the major organ systems, much less precision in coding is likely. Major differences may exist between the way a set of certificates are filled out by different physicians or coded by different nosologists.

Since it must be recognized that observation bias is always present in coding death certificates, it follows that in analyzing mortality data caution must be exercised in dealing with positive findings. At a minimum, the certificates for persons with an apparent excess disease must be examined to determine the likelihood that the excess has arisen from coding inconsistencies. No such false excesses were detected in the B. F. Goodrich data.

2. Data Analysis and Results

Data analysis was carried out using a computer program developed to analyze data from cohort studies.[16] Since partial follow-up was conducted through the Social Security Administration, there was an under-ascertainment of deaths prior to around 1940. Therefore, follow-up was started as of January 1, 1940. Persons who had worked at least 5 years and who were actively employed on or after 1/1/40 were included.

a. Mortality Patterns among Entire Cohort

Among the cohort of 13,571 white male union members, 5079 deaths were observed and 6090.6 were expected (Table 6.1). The SMR was $100 \times (5079/6090.6) = 83$. The two highest SMRs were for bladder cancer (122) and leukemia (129). The SMR of 93 for all cancers was higher than the SMR of 83 for all causes. SMRs less than 80 were seen for all causes of death other than cancer or cardiovascular disease.

In Table 6.2, patterns of mortality from all causes are presented according to age and calendar year.[4] The ratio of observed to expected deaths (SMR/100) is presented for simplicity, but for brevity the ratio is referred to as the SMR. As reported elsewhere,[14,15] the SMR approaches 1.0 as the population ages. The time trend in the SMR from 0.7 in 1940—49 to 0.9 in 1970—74 is simply a reflection of this aging of the population: the age-specific pattern is similar within each decade group but the 1970—74 stratum is heavily weighted with older persons.

As seen in Table 6.3, there is not much association of the SMR with age or year started work. The ratio of 1.4 in persons who started work at age 45 or above and before 1920 is relatively high, but must be interpreted with caution. Since follow-up did not start until 1940, these persons were all at least 65 when follow-up started.

In Table 6.4, SMRs are presented according to years worked and latency. Since the cohort was comprised only of persons who worked at least 5 years, no information is available for persons who worked fewer than 5 years or for latency less than 5 years. The SMRs along the lower diagonal largely reflect the mortality experience of the active work force: these persons died no later than 5 years after they stopped working; many died while actively employed. It can be seen that in each of the cells of this lower diagonal, the SMR is between 0.6 and 0.8.

The SMRs in the next diagonal to the right tend to lie between 0.9 and 1.1. Each of these SMRs is higher than that in the preceding latency stratum and higher than that in the succeeding years worked stratum. This no doubt is simply a reflection of the retirement pattern of healthy and unhealthy workers: those who are unhealthy (for any reason) retire and have a higher risk of dying within 5 to 10 years than do those who continue to work. This cannot simply be an age phenomenon, since as seen in Table 6.2, the SMR for death from all causes above age 65 is only 0.9.

The trend in the SMR with years worked (range 0.7 to 0.9) is less than the trend with latency (range 0.6 to 1.3). For persons who worked at least 25 years, there is a tendency toward excess mortality after retirement; for persons who worked fewer than 25 years, no such tendency is apparent. It is possible that part of this difference may be due to observation bias. Persons who worked relatively short periods of time were followed for mortality mainly through the SSA. To the extent that deaths were under-ascertained by the SSA, this under-ascertainment would mainly affect those who worked the fewest number of years.

Since over 50% of deaths are due to cardiovascular disease (circulatory and cerebrovascular), the patterns of mortality for all causes heavily reflect the patterns for cardiovascular disease.

In Tables 6.5 to 6.7, patterns of mortality for all cancers are presented. In comparison to the patterns for all causes of death as presented in Table 6.2, there is no trend in the association of the SMR for all cancer with age at death, and consequently no trend with calendar time (Table 6.5). In comparing Tables 6.3 and 6.6, the patterns according to age and year started working are similar.

In comparing Tables 6.4 and 6.7, patterns of mortality according to years worked and latency, there are some similarities and some differences. The cells in the lowest diagonal tend to have SMRs lower than in neighboring cells, although there is more variability for all cancers than for all causes. There are some relatively high (although absolutely weak) SMRs in the low years worked — latency cells as well as in the high.

Table 6.2
OBSERVED/EXPECTED DEATHS FROM ALL CAUSES AND RATIO OF OBSERVED TO EXPECTED DEATHS AMONG 13,571 WHITE MALE RUBBER WORKERS ACCORDING TO AGE AND CALENDAR YEAR

Observed/expected deaths

Age	Calendar year				
	1940—49	1950—59	1960—69	1970—74	Total
<45	113/164	106/146	53/73	5/8	277/391
45—54	147/254	206/276	233/280	66/80	652/890
55—64	194/295	433/542	486/574	153/223	1266/1634
65—74	121/145	448/484	787/873	306/373	1662/1875
≥75	25/21	162/174	586/637	449/469	1222/1301
Total	600/879	1355/1622	2145/2437	979/1153	5079/6091

Ratio of observed to expected deaths

Age	1940—49	1950—59	1960—69	1970—74	Total
<45	0.7	0.7	0.7	0.6	0.7
45—54	0.6	0.8	0.8	0.8	0.7
55—64	0.7	0.8	0.9	0.7	0.8
65—74	0.8	0.9	0.9	0.8	0.9
≥75	1.2	0.9	0.9	1.0	0.9
Total	0.7	0.8	0.9	0.9	0.8

Table 6.3
RATIO OF OBSERVED TO EXPECTED DEATHS FROM ALL CAUSES ACCORDING TO AGE AND CALENDAR YEAR OF STARTING WORK

Age started work	Calendar year started work				
	<1920	1920—29	1930—39	≥1940	Total
<25	0.8	0.7	0.7	0.7	0.7
25—34	1.0	0.8	0.7	0.8	0.8
35—44	0.9	0.9	1.0	1.0	0.9
≥45	1.4	0.7	0.8	0.9	0.8
Total	0.9	0.8	0.8	0.9	0.8

In Tables 6.8 and 6.9, patterns of mortality for external causes (accidents, poisoning and violence) are presented. There is no indication that mortality from these causes has occurred to excess among members of this cohort. Further, it is unlikely that long term exposures to substances used in industry would lead to death from one of these causes. As seen in Table 6.8, the SMR for these causes is quite low below the age of

Table 6.4

RATIO OF OBSERVED TO EXPECTED DEATHS FROM ALL CAUSES ACCORDING TO YEARS WORKED AND YEARS SINCE WORK STARTED (LATENCY)[a]

Years worked	Years since work started (latency)											
	5—9	10—14	15—19	20—24	25—29	30—34	35—39	40—44	45—49	50—54	55 +	Total
5—9	0.8	0.9	0.8	0.7	0.6	0.6	1.0	—				0.7
10—14		0.7	0.9	1.1	0.8	0.7	0.9	(1.4)	—			0.8
15—19			0.6	1.1	0.8	0.8	0.8	1.0	(1.1)	—		0.7
20—24				0.7	1.1	0.9	1.1	1.0	0.7	(0.6)	—	0.9
25—29					0.7	1.2	1.1	1.1	1.2	1.3	—	0.9
30—34						0.6	1.0	1.1	1.2	1.4	(0.9)	0.9
35—39							0.7	0.9	1.1	1.1	1.5	0.9
40—44								0.7	0.8	0.6	1.3	0.9
45 +									0.7	0.7	1.1	0.8
Total	0.8	0.7	0.6	0.8	0.8	0.8	0.9	1.0	1.0	1.2	1.3	0.8

[a]
— Fewer than four deaths expected.
( ) Four to ten deaths expected.

Table 6.5
RATIO OF OBSERVED TO EXPECTED DEATHS FROM ALL CANCERS ACCORDING TO AGE AND CALENDAR YEAR

Observed/expected deaths

Age	\multicolumn{5}{c}{Calendar year}
	1940—49	1950—59	1960—69	1970—74	Total
<45	17/15	20/18	7/10	2/1	46/44
45—54	27/34	32/46	54/52	13/17	126/149
55—64	36/44	85/107	105/121	35/55	261/327
65—74	22/23	88/86	168/171	67/82	345/362
≥75	3/7	19/23	106/84	80/69	208/183
Total	105/123	244/280	440/438	197/224	986/1065

Ratio of observed to expected deaths

Age	1940—49	1950—59	1960—69	1970—74	Total
<45	1.1	1.1	0.7	—	1.1
45—54	0.8	0.7	1.0	0.8	0.9
55—64	0.8	0.8	0.9	0.6	0.8
65—74	1.0	1.0	1.0	0.8	1.0
≥75	—	0.8	1.3	1.2	1.1
Total	0.9	0.9	1.0	0.9	0.9

Table 6.6
RATIO OF OBSERVED TO EXPECTED DEATHS FROM ALL CANCERS ACCORDING TO AGE AND CALENDAR YEAR OF STARTING WORK[a]

Age started work	\multicolumn{5}{c}{Calendar year started work}
	<1920	1920—29	1930—39	≥1940	Total
<25	1.0	0.7	0.7	1.0	0.8
25—34	1.0	0.9	0.8	0.9	0.9
35—44	0.9	1.2	1.0	1.0	1.1
≥45	—	1.0	1.0	0.9	1.0
Total	1.0	0.9	0.9	1.0	0.9

[a] — Fewer than four deaths expected.

65; above this age there is only a slight deficit. The pattern of mortality in Table 6.9 shows little association with years worked or with latency. However, as with all causes, all cardiovascular diseases and all cancers, the SMRs in the lowest diagonal (the SMRs for active workers) tend to be lower than for their neighbors.

In Tables 6.10 to 6.12, patterns of SMRs for death from leukemia are presented. As seen in Table 6.1, leukemia has the highest SMR in the cohort (129). As will be discussed later, it is likely that some of the substances used in the rubber industry in the past were causes of leukemia.

Table 6.7

RATIO OF OBSERVED TO EXPECTED DEATHS FROM ALL CANCERS ACCORDING TO YEARS WORKED AND YEARS SINCE WORK STARTED (LATENCY)[a]

Years worked	Years since work started (latency)										Total
	5—9	10—14	15—19	20—24	25—29	30—34	35—39	40—44	45—49	50—54	
5—9	1.1	(0.6)	1.2	0.8	0.9	0.4	(0.0)				0.8
10—14		1.0	1.4	1.3	0.9	0.6	(1.4)	—			1.0
15—19			0.6	0.9	0.5	0.8	0.9	(1.4)	—		0.8
20—24				0.9	0.9	1.1	1.0	(0.9)	(0.7)	—	0.9
25—29					0.8	1.1	1.2	0.9	(1.6)	—	1.0
30—34						0.9	0.9	1.2	1.3	(0.8)	1.0
35—39							0.7	1.2	1.1	1.5	0.9
40—44								0.8	0.7	1.6	0.9
45 +									(1.2)	(1.3)	1.2
Total	1.1	0.9	0.8	0.9	0.8	0.9	0.9	1.0	1.1	1.4	0.9

[a] — Fewer than four deaths expected.
( ) Four to ten deaths expected.

Table 6.8
OBSERVED/EXPECTED DEATHS FROM EXTERNAL CAUSES ACCORDING TO AGE AND CALENDAR YEAR

Observed/expected deaths

Age	Calendar year				
	1940—49	1950—59	1960—69	1970—74	Total
<45	31/50	29/47	12/21	1/3	73/121
45—64	28/54	40/67	40/69	9/24	117/214
≥65	10/8	21/25	34/48	24/24	89/105
Total	69/112	90/139	86/138	34/51	279/440

Ratio of observed to expected deaths

Age	1940—49	1950—59	1960—69	1970—74	Total
<45	0.6	0.6	0.6	—	0.6
45—64	0.5	0.6	0.6	0.4	0.6
≥65	1.3	0.8	0.7	1.0	0.9
Total	0.6	0.7	0.6	0.7	0.6

Table 6.9
RATIO OF OBSERVED TO EXPECTED DEATHS FROM EXTERNAL CAUSES ACCORDING TO YEARS WORKED AND YEARS SINCE WORK STARTED (LATENCY)[a]

Years worked	Years since work started (latency)									
	5—9	10—14	15—19	20—24	25—29	30—34	35—39	40—44	45 +	Total
5—9	0.6	0.4	0.6	0.5	(0.7)	—	—			0.6
10—14		0.5	(0.8)	(0.8)	(0.9)	—	—	—		0.7
15—19			0.6	(1.2)	(0.9)	—	—	—	—	0.7
20—24				0.6	(0.7)	(1.0)	—	—	—	0.7
25—29					0.6	(0.9)	(0.7)	—	—	0.6
30—34						0.5	(1.2)	(0.4)	—	0.6
35—39							0.5	(0.8)	(2.2)	0.9
40 +								(0.5)	(0.7)	0.6
Total	0.6	0.5	0.6	0.7	0.6	0.6	0.8	0.6	(1.0)	0.6

[a]   — Fewer than four deaths expected.
      ( ) Four to ten deaths expected.

As seen in Table 6.10, the excess of leukemia was seen in persons dying in all calendar periods and in all ages under 75. There is therefore no evidence that the effects of any causal exposures have disappeared, although the excess in 1970—74 is modest. As seen in Table 6.11, no excess is seen in persons who started working after 1934, suggesting that if the association is causal, the responsible substance is no longer being used. It seems unlikely that this lack of an excess among these workers is due to their

Table 6.10
OBSERVED/EXPECTED DEATHS FROM LEUKEMIA AND RATIO OF OBSERVED TO EXPECTED DEATHS ACCORDING TO AGE AND CALENDAR YEAR

Observed/expected deaths

| Age | Calendar year | | | |
	1940—59	1960—69	1970—74	Total
<55	6/6.0	5/2.9	0/0.9	11/9.8
55—64	9/5.3	4/4.1	2/1.6	15/11.0
65—74	5/4.0	11/6.7	5/2.8	21/13.5
≥75	0/1.2	5/4.0	3/3.2	8/8.4
Total	20/16.5	25/17.7	10/8.5	55/42.7

Ratio of observed to expected deaths

<55	1.0	1.7	—	1.1
55—64	1.7	1.0	1.3	1.4
65—74	1.3	1.6	1.8	1.6
≥75	—	1.3	0.9	1.0
Total	1.2	1.4	1.2	1.3

Table 6.11
OBSERVED/EXPECTED DEATHS FROM LEUKEMIA AND RATIO OF OBSERVED TO EXPECTED DEATHS ACCORDING TO AGE AND CALENDAR YEAR OF STARTING WORK

Observed/expected deaths

| Age started work | Calendar year started work | | | |
	<1925	1925—34	>1935	Total
<25	11/3.7	7/4.0	2/3.3	20/11.0
25—34	6/7.8	7/6.3	4/3.2	17/17.3
≥35	4/3.5	11/5.0	3/5.9	18/14.4
Total	21/15.0	25/15.3	9/12.4	55/42.7

Ratio of observed to expected deaths

<25	3.0	1.8	0.6	1.8
25—34	0.8	1.1	1.3	1.0
≥35	1.1	2.2	0.5	1.3
Total	1.4	1.6	0.7	1.3

Table 6.12
OBSERVED/EXPECTED DEATHS FROM LEUKEMIA
AND RATIO OF OBSERVED TO EXPECTED DEATHS
ACCORDING TO YEARS WORKED AND LATENCY

Observed/expected deaths

Years worked	Latency					
	5—14	15—24	25—34	35—44	≥45	Total
5—14	2/4.1	1/2.4	0/2.3	1/0.6		4/9.4
15—24		8/6.3	4/2.7	3/1.4	0/0.3	15/10.7
25—34			15/8.1	5/4.0	2/1.3	22/13.4
35—44				6/5.3	5/3.3	11/8.6
≥45					3/0.6	3/0.6
Total	2/4.1	9/8.7	19/13.1	15/11.3	10/5.5	55/42.7

Ratio of observed to expected deaths

	5—14	15—24	25—34	35—44	≥45	Total
5—14	0.5	0.4	—	—		0.4
15—24		1.3	1.5	2.1	—	1.4
25—34			1.9	1.3	1.5	1.6
35—44				1.1	1.5	1.3
≥45					—	—
Total	0.5	1.0	1.5	1.3	1.7	1.3

being relatively young, since as seen in Table 6.10, the excess is present in persons aged less than 55 and no excess is seen in those over age 74.

Another possibility for the lack of an excess in persons who started working after 1934 is that they have not been exposed for a long enough period of time. As seen in Table 6.12, no excess of leukemia was seen in persons who worked fewer than 15 years; also, the excess was not seen until at least 25 years of latency. While this may account for some of the lack of excess among persons who started working in later years, many of these persons worked for at least 15 years and were followed for at least 25 years.

Since no excess of death from leukemia was seen in persons who started working after 1934, analysis was limited to persons who started working before 1935. As seen in Table 6.13, the excess is seen essentially only in persons who worked 15 years or more and who were followed 25 years or more. Excess deaths occurred among persons in the "active" cells (the lower diagonal) as well as in the "retired" cells.

The above patterns of mortality were given for members of the entire cohort of 13,571 workers. Since this was a very heterogeneous work force, it is unlikely that all workers shared common exposures. Indeed, if analyses are limited to persons who worked in specific departments, excesses of specific cancers are seen.[1-4] The main difficulty is size: even though this is a large cohort, a much smaller number of workers shared common work patterns. Fortunately, few diseases occurred to high excess. Therefore, any department-disease associations are based on relatively small numbers and are quite unstable.

b. Mortality Patterns According to Mode of Follow-Up

As indicated, it is desirable in a cohort study to determine the vital status of each

Table 6.13
OBSERVED/EXPECTED DEATHS FROM LEUKEMIA AND RATIO OF OBSERVED TO EXPECTED DEATHS ACCORDING TO YEARS WORKED AND LATENCY; PERSONS INCLUDED ARE ONLY THOSE WHO STARTED WORK BEFORE 1935

Observed/expected deaths

Years worked	Latency					
	5—14	15—24	25—34	35—44	≥45	Total
5—14	0/0.9	0/0.5	0/0.8	1/0.4		1/2.6
15—24		5/3.5	4/1.7	3/1.4	0/0.3	12/6.9
25—34			13/6.3	5/3.9	2/1.3	20/11.5
35—44				5/5.3	5/3.3	10/8.6
≥45					3/0.6	3/0.6
Total	0/0.9	5/4.0	17/8.8	14/11.0	10/5.5	46/30.2

Ratio of observed to expected deaths

5—14	—	—	—	—		0.4
15—24		1.4	2.4	2.1	—	1.7
25—34			2.1	1.3	1.5	1.7
35—44				0.9	1.5	1.2
≥45					—	—
Total	—	1.3	1.9	1.3	1.8	1.5

individual as of the common closing date of follow-up. If persons are lost-to-follow-up, there is uncertainty as to their mortality patterns after loss. There is concern that persons who are lost may have work-related diseases that lead to excess deaths.

It was possible to examine the question of completeness of follow-up in the B. F. Goodrich rubber worker data. As indicated, death certificates were available through the company for persons who died while actively employed or while covered by a death benefit plan. Among the 13,571 employees who were followed for 253,000 person-years while under follow-up by the Company,[1] 3783 deaths were observed for a SMR of 86 (Table 6.14). Among the 4164 employees who terminated employment prior to death or to receiving vested rights, there were 88,000 person-years of follow-up and 1199 deaths for a SMR of 73. As seen in Table 6.14, the SMRs for the various categories of causes of death are similar for the two periods of follow-up.

While these data provide no support for the concern that terminated employees have an abnormally high death rate following termination, they must be interpreted with caution. Since follow-up for the terminated employees was conducted through the SSA, any under-ascertainment will affect this group exclusively. However, fairly substantial numbers of deaths would have to be missed by the SSA in order to lead to a total misrepresentation of the SMRs among terminated employees. With respect to all causes, 214 deaths among terminated employees would have to have been missed if this true SMR were 86 ([86/73] [1199] − 1199). With respect to all cancers, for which there is specific concern, there is no evidence for even a relative excess among those followed through the SSA. It does not seem likely that the SSA would selectively under-ascertain death from cancer, especially since persons with cancer tend to die in medical care facilities.

c. Comparison Between External and Internal Controls

In the initial analysis of data on B. F. Goodrich rubber workers, the numbers of deaths observed from specific causes were compared to the numbers expected, based on U.S. mortality rates.[1] Subsequently, supplemental data on cancer were obtained from Akron-area tumor registries.[3] Rates of cancer within the cohort were made by computing age-standardized cancer morbidity rates for different groups of workers. In the initial analysis indirect standardization was used; in the second analysis the rates were directly standardized.

In Table 6.15, the results of the two analyses are compared for stomach and intestinal cancer among men who made rubber. In the initial mortality analysis, twice as many of these cancers were observed among rubber makers vs. those expected based on U.S. mortality rates. Among all other rubber workers, slight deficits of these cancers were seen. Since rubber makers were somewhat older than the other workers,[1] a question could be raised as to whether the excess seen in them was simply due to age differences relative to other workers.

In the internal comparison, age-standardized rates were computed by the direct method. Therefore, the standardized rates for each of the cancers is directly comparable between rubber makers and the residual workers. By definition, the rate ratio in the residual workers is 1.0. As can be seen, the ratio of the two obs/exp ratios (SMRs) is essentially the same as the directly standardized rate ratio.

Such comparability is frequently seen in comparing the results of indirect and direct standardization. An advantage of the SMR is that it indicates that the occurrence of stomach and intestinal cancer is in excess among the rubber makers. If only the internal comparisons were available, it would not be known whether the rates among the rubber makers were in excess or the rates in the residual workers were in deficit.

In this example, at least, indirect and direct standardization led to essentially the same measure of association between rubber making and stomach and intestinal cancer. While in other circumstances such similarity may not result, indirect standardization should not be dismissed simply because of theoretical objections.

d. Mortality Patterns Among Sub-Groups of Cohort

In the example of indirect vs. direct standardization, the rates of stomach and intestinal cancer among men who worked in the rubber making departments were compared to the rates among all other men. It is usual in studies of occupational groups to separate the entire cohort into its component parts.

There are essentially three strategies that can be used in analyzing cohort data where the members of the cohort have worked in more than one work area: (1) count a person once — in the work area in which he worked the longest; (2) count a person in each of the work areas in which he worked; (3) count a person in each of the work areas in which he worked, but stratify all persons in a given work area as to length of time worked.

Strategy one has the advantage of counting each person only once; therefore mutually exclusive subgroups of a cohort can be defined. Also, there is a tendency to exclude persons who worked only a short time in a given area and therefore such persons would not dilute any association between work in that area and disease. However, some persons with considerable experience in two or more work areas may not be counted in the area which contributed the most to his terminal illness.

Strategy two has the advantage that everyone who ever worked in a specific area is

Table 6.14
NUMBERS OF DEATHS OBSERVED AMONG RUBBER WORKERS AND RATIOS OF OBSERVED TO EXPECTED ACCORDING TO TWO PERIODS OF FOLLOW-UP[a]

Cause of death	Observed deaths		Observed/ expected[b]	
	A	B	A	B
All causes[c]	3783	1199	0.86	0.73
All cancer	728	252	0.98	0.83
CNS vascular	352	141	0.90	0.96
Circulatory	1873	572	0.89	0.68
External	206	72	0.65	0.56
All other causes	624	162	0.70	0.50

[a] Period A: Person-years accumulated while actively working or while retired with death benefits. Deaths ascertained from company records.
Period B: Person-years accumulated after leaving employ of company. Deaths ascertained from Social Security Administration.

[b] Expected numbers based on 5-year age-time specific mortality rates for U.S. white males.

[c] Excludes 97 deaths of unknown cause.

Table 6.15
MORBIDITY FROM STOMACH AND INTESTINAL CANCER AMONG RUBBER MAKERS AND OTHER RUBBER WORKERS[a,b]

Type of cancer	Work area	External comparison (Deaths 1940—1974.5)			Internal comparison (All cases 1940—1976.5)		
		Observed	Expected	Obs/exp	N	Rate[b]	Ratio
Stomach	Rubber making	12	5.7	2.1	13	63	2.2
	Residual	82	86.1	1.0	92	29	1.0
Intestine	Rubber making	13	6.5	2.0	17	78	2.0
	Residual	86	94.5	0.9	122	38	1.0

[a] Expected deaths based on age-time-cause specific mortality rates among U.S. white males.

[b] Standardized by the direct method to the age distribution of all 13,571 rubber workers.

counted. The disadvantage is that persons are counted more than once, but they can only die once. If there is some work area which tends to some disease and if there is some second work area in which persons of the first work area tend also to work, there may arise a false impression that the second area is also a dangerous place in which to work.

Strategy three has some of the good features of the other two strategies but also some of the bad. A person is counted in as many work areas as he has worked, and thus his entire work history can be utilized. However, while he still can die only once, his death will be counted in each of his work areas.

In using strategy three, a person enters follow-up for a given work area only when he enters that area. However, he continues in follow-up even if he changes to another area. His "years worked" are specific to the years in a specific area. Data can be computed as illustrated in Tables 6.2 to 6.4. As indicated, such a person will be counted more than once. However, if he works only 1 year in one department (A) but 20 years in a second (B), his expected numbers (and observed death) will be in the <5 strata for department A and in the 20 to 24 stratum for department B. If there is an association between work and some cause of death, it is most likely to be detected in persons who have worked some minimum number of years. An erroneous appearance of an excess in the department A would arise only if persons who work 20+ years in department B are also likely to work less than 5 years in department A. This can usually be examined by stratifying persons who worked in department A into those who worked 20 or more years in department B and those who did not. If no excess is seen among persons who worked in department A but not in B, one would conclude that working in department B was simply a confounding factor for some of the persons who worked in department A.

In the rubber worker data, initial analyses were done according to strategy one and strategy two. The results are presented in Table 6.16. As can be seen, the results tend to be similar, although there is not much variation in the SMRs for these heterogeneous groups. Consider the data for all cancers: where the SMR for "usual" is low, the SMR for "ever" is higher. This results simply because of the dilution of "usual" workers with persons whose SMR is closer to the average for the entire group.

Analyses using strategy three are in progress.[4]

e. Maximum Number of Deaths Expected

It has been suggested that as a cohort ages and more and more of its members die, the expected number of deaths approaches and can go no higher than the total number in the cohort.[17] For example, in a cohort of 100 persons, the expected number of deaths should be no greater than 100. While this is certainly true for the observed number, this must not necessarily be true for the expected number.

There were 131 rubber workers who started working before 1910 and who were still working in 1940. As of 7/1/1974, 117 of these persons were deceased, 13 were still alive and 1 was lost-to-follow-up. Based on U.S. mortality rates, the expected number of deaths was 136.1. The SMR was $100 \times 117/136.1$ or 86.

Such a result is to be expected when any healthy group is followed until most of its members are deceased. In any given year, there is a tendency for fewer persons to die than expected. Since the SMR is simply the sum of the observed divided by the sum of the expected for each year, it must be that when the observed number reaches the total number in the cohort, the expected number can be greater than the total number. Therefore, it does not follow that as a cohort ages, the amount of information contained in the SMR decreases.

3. Interpretation of Data from Rubber Workers

In the tables in this chapter no measures of stability (p-values or confidence limits) are presented. I find little utility to such measures when evaluating the association between many work areas (200 +) and many causes of death (50 +). For reasons discussed above and in Chapter 5, simple measures of statistical significance tend to be of limited value in interpreting these associations. Further, much inspection of the data and combination of groups of workers was needed in the analysis of these data. The process is much more intuitive than statistical.

Because of the intuitive nature of much of this and other epidemiologic analyses, data interpretation must take into account other data sources. Data on other rubber workers that are analyzed by other investigators are subject to other sources of bias and error. If, in spite of these perturbations, similar associations are seen, belief as to the causal nature of the association is enhanced. An illustration of such consistency is presented in Tables 5.3 and 5.4.

The excess occurrence of leukemia among rubber workers is one that probably is causal. In two studies the excess appears to be highest among persons with solvent exposure.[3,18] As seen in Table 6.12, there is an association with year started working. As seen in Table 6.13, there is an association both with years worked and with latency.

However, the substance responsible for the excess has not been identified. A primary suspect is benzene, but benzene was not used extensively prior to 1935.[3] Also, the cell type that predominates among rubber workers (lymphatic) differs from that among benzene workers (myeloid).[19] Thus, even though a causal association with rubber work can be inferred, it does not follow that a means of prevention is at hand.

In studies like that of the rubber workers, a number of associations will be seen that cannot be explained.[3] Whether these associations are causal may never be known. However, an understanding of the reason for an apparent excess of some diseases is not a prerequisite for action to be taken in reducing exposure to potentially hazardous substances. At some point it becomes more reasonable to act as if work in some area is hazardous than to wait for further information. Since there always will be differing opinions as to where this point is, data interpretation is more than a scientific or statistical process. Further, rather than reducing exposure to one substance, it is usually more logical to reduce overall exposure in a work area. Only through such general improvement in environmental conditions can there be a reduction in work-related illness.

III. PROPORTIONAL MORTALITY STUDIES (SPMR STUDIES)

In evaluating patterns of mortality among a group of employed persons, it is preferable to obtain vital status information on the entire cohort so that comparison of rates can be carried out. Frequently, however, one may have access simply to the death certificates on a group of workers. If the time and money needed to follow all workers are not available, a standardized proportional mortality analysis of the death certificates can provide valuable information.

A. Procedure

Death certificates are accumulated and coded as described earlier in this chapter. Analysis is carried out as described in Chapter 4. Rather than computing expected numbers of deaths on the basis of age-time-cause specific mortality rates, expected numbers are computed on the basis of age-time-cause specific proportions or percentages.

Analyses may be carried out in a manner analagous to that used for standardized mortality ratio analyses. The deceased persons can be stratified on the basis of departmental work experience (e.g., usual, ever, or years worked in a department), on the basis of year or age started working, or on the basis of years worked and latency.

There is no analogue to the HWE in a proportional mortality analysis, since by definition the total number of deaths expected must be equal to the total number of deaths observed. However, the HWE probably has some influence on cause-specific proportional mortality ratios. SMRs for all cancers tend to be higher than SMRs for all other causes, usually by 10 to 20%. Therefore, even if there is no absolute excess of cancer among a group of deceased persons, for methodologic reasons an excess of 10 to 20% might be expected. Note that in the realm of rate ratios, this is a very weak association.

Also, SPMRs tend to be more interpretable for uncommon causes of death than for common causes. If the rate of some uncommon disease such as lung cancer is increased by, say, 200%, the SMR and the SPMR will each reflect this increase. However, if a common illness such as circulatory disease is increased by 200%, the SMR will still reflect this increase, while the SPMR will be increased considerably less. Also, whereas SMRs for two or more causes are essentially independent of each other, SPMRs for two or more causes are interdependent, since the sum of the expected numbers must equal the sum of the observed numbers.

In spite of these limitations to SPMR analyses, they are most useful and provide information that usually differs little from that obtained in an SMR analysis. It is especially instructive to do SPMR and SMR analyses on the same data, so as to evaluate interpretation of the results of these two methods of analysis.

B. Example — Rubber Workers

Consider again the data in Table 6.1. In assessing whether a specific cause of death is in excess, one might look only at causes for which the SMR is greater than 100. If this criterion is used, only leukemia and cancers of the stomach, large intestine, and bladder are in excess among the entire group of rubber workers. However, it might be argued that because of the HWE (or because of some other bias), SMRs greater than the "all-causes" SMR should be considered to be in excess. Intuitively, one assesses such excess by dividing each cause-specific SMR by the all-causes SMR to obtain a "corrected" SMR (CSMR).[20]

The results of such a division are illustrated in Table 6.17. In Column I are the same SMRs as in Table 6.1 (note that the SMRs differ slightly because the analyses were carried out at different times). In Column II are the CSMRs. CSMRs less than 100 are seen only for diseases other than cancer or cardiovascular disease. In Column III are the SPMRs from a proportional mortality analysis. By definition the all-cause CSMR and the SPMR are 1.00.

It can be seen that the CSMR and the SPMR for the several causes illustrated are similar. Part of the similarity no doubt is due to the relatively weak associations between disease and working in the rubber industry. However, under any of the three methods used to compute expected numbers, one would wish to investigate further death from bladder cancer and the lymphatic and hematopoietic cancers.

There is one tendency in Table 6.17 that may be of interest. For diseases of old persons, e.g., bladder cancer and stroke, the CSMR is higher than the SPMR. For diseases of young persons, e.g., brain cancer and external causes of death, the SPMR is higher than the CSMR. Whether this tendency is a general property of the CSMR and the SPMR is unknown. If it is a general property, it no doubt results from the way the weights differ between a SMR computation and SPMR computation, i.e., person-years vs. numbers of deaths.

C. Example — Vinyl Chloride Workers

In 1974, three cases of angiosarcoma of the liver among vinyl chloride workers were

Table 6.16
STANDARDIZED MORTALITY RATIOS (AND OBSERVED DEATHS) ACCORDING TO PLANT DIVISION IN WHICH EMPLOYEES EVER AND USUALLY WORKED[a]

Division	All causes		All cancers	
	Ever	Usual	Ever	Usual
"Laid Off"	—	81 (319)	—	69 (44)
Chemical	74 (161)	74 (68)	85 (32)	80 (13)
Aerospace	74 (711)	81 (282)	92 (155)	89 (55)
Tires	79 (1968)	81 (1345)	92 (397)	93 (265)
Industrial products	76 (1600)	81 (796)	84 (309)	94 (159)
Services	83 (2238)	84 (1638)	90 (405)	94 (305)
Rubber reclaim	75 (313)	72 (93)	94 (68)	100 (22)
Processing	79 (833)	87 (538)	98 (177)	111 (117)
Total	—	82 (5079)	—	94 (980)

[a]   Data differ slightly from those presented in Table 6.1.

Table 6.17
NUMBER OF DEATHS OBSERVED AMONG RUBBER WORKERS AND RATIOS OF OBSERVED TO EXPECTED ACCORDING TO THREE METHODS

Cause of death	Observed deaths	Observed/expected[b]		
		I	II	III
All causes	4982[a]	0.82	1.00	1.00
All cancer	980	0.94	1.17	1.17
Digestive	364	0.98	1.22	1.21
Bladder	48	1.22	1.52	1.45
Brain	20	0.80	1.00	1.10
Lymphatic and hematopoietic	106	1.13	1.42	1.44
CNS vascular	493	0.91	1.13	1.07
Circulatory	2445	0.83	1.03	1.01
External	278	0.62	0.77	0.86
All other causes	786	0.65	0.74	0.77

[a]   Excludes 97 deaths of unknown cause.

[b]   I   Expected numbers based on 5-year age-time specific mortality rates for U.S. white males (SMR/100).

II   Expected ratios in I have been divided by 0.82 (all causes SMR/100) and by 0.98 to correct for 97 deaths of unknown cause (CSMR/100).

III   Expected numbers based on 5-year age-time specific proportional mortality ratios for U.S. white males (SPMR/100).

reported.[21] Later in the same year, the results of two epidemiologic studies were reported. In one, a standardized proportional mortality analysis was conducted of the causes of death among 161 deceased persons, most of whom had worked at the same plant as the three with angiosarcoma.[22] In the second, a standardized mortality ratio

Table 6.18
OBSERVED AND EXPECTED DEATHS
AMONG VINYL CHLORIDE WORKERS IN
A PROPORTIONAL MORTALITY STUDY[a]

Cause of death	Observed	Expected	SPMR[b]
All causes	161	161.0	100
All cancer	41	27.9	150
Digestive	13	8.3	160
Liver and biliary	8	0.7	1100
Lung	13	7.9	160
Brain	5	1.2	420
Other	10	10.5	95
CNS vascular	8	9.5	80
Circulatory	66	68.6	96
External	22	24.5	90
All other causes	24	30.5	79

[a] Expected numbers based on proportional mortality ratios for United States white males.

[b] SPMR = Standardized proportional mortality ratio = 100 × observed/expected.

analysis was conducted on the mortality among 8384 men who had worked with vinyl chloride, including those at the same plant as above.[23] Among these 8384 workers were 352 who had died, including most of the 161 included in the above report.

In Table 6.18 are presented the results of the SPMR study. A 50% excess of cancer was seen, which was due entirely to cancers of the liver, the lung, and the brain. In Table 6.19 are presented the results of the SMR study. As compared to the general population, there was essentially no excess of cancer. However, the CSMR was (102/75) × 100 or 136. There were large excesses of cancers of the liver and of the brain. For respiratory cancer, while the SMR was close to 100, the CSMR was 140.

Thus the two studies reported similar results, even though one was smaller and based simply on a SPMR analysis. In this study an analysis according to age and year of death of persons with cancer was also done (Table 6.20). As can be seen, while there is no trend with age at death, there is a steady increase in the SPMR with year of death. This suggests that many more persons will die from cancer because of exposure to vinyl chloride.

The judgment as to whether the excesses of specific causes of death are likely to be causal is based on reason rather than any statistical significance. There can be little doubt that vinyl chloride (or some closely related compound) is responsible for the angiosarcoma. This disease was extremely rare before it was discovered among vinyl chloride workers. The rate ratio among vinyl chloride workers must be in the 1000s. The disease occurred mainly in the men who worked for many years (10 +) cleaning the reactors; these men accumulated a high dosage of exposure to vinyl chloride. This was so after the first three cases of angiosarcoma were identified.

With respect to cancers of the brain and of the lung, a causal interpretation of the association is not possible at the moment. Both are relatively common cancers and are based on much smaller rate ratios. The cause of most of lung cancer is known, and the excess seen here could conceivably be due to cigarette smoking. The cause of most of brain cancer is not known.

It is mainly of scientific interest whether vinyl chloride exposure leads to brain or

Table 6.19
OBSERVED AND EXPECTED DEATHS AMONG VINYL CHLORIDE WORKERS IN A MORTALITY STUDY[a]

Cause of death	Observed	Expected	SMR
All causes	352	467.3	75
All cancer	79	77.2	102
Digestive	19	21.7	88
Liver	7	1.7	412
Respiratory	25	23.9	105
Brain	7	2.5	280
Other	10	9.3	108
CNS vascular	13	24.5	57
Circulatory	142	178.8	79
External	52	91.7	57
All other causes	66	95.1	69

[a] Expected numbers based on mortality rates for United States white males.

Table 6.20
OBSERVED AND EXPECTED DEATHS FROM ALL CANCERS AMONG VINYL CHLORIDE WORKERS IN A PROPORTIONAL MORTALITY STUDY ACCORDING TO AGE AND YEAR OF DEATH

Characteristic	Category	Observed	Expected	SPMR
Age of death	<50	11	7.6	140
	50—59	17	8.1	210
	≥60	13	12.2	110
Year of death	<1965	12	11.4	110
	1965—69	10	7.3	140
	≥1970	19	9.2	210

lung cancer. Exposure must be reduced because of its highly likely role in causing angiosarcoma. If some lung and brain cancer are also prevented, so much the better.

IV. CASE-CONTROL STUDIES WITHIN A COHORT

On occasion, personnel records may be available for a cohort of employed persons, but it may be too expensive to review all of the records to determine the work history of each person. Some sample of the records is selected to be reviewed. Since a primary interest in such review is to determine association between work and disease, priority is given to reviewing the work histories of persons with one or more diseases of interest. For purposes of comparison, the work histories of "controls" are also determined.

A. Procedure
In this discussion, it is assumed that mortality data for the entire cohort are available. Initial analyses proceed as described in Section II of this chapter, including Tables 6.1 to 6.13. If one or more causes of death are found to be in excess and if there is

concern that occupational factors may be responsible, further information on the work histories of these persons should be assembled.

The cases are persons who have died of the disease of interest. Several possibilities exist as to who may be selected as the controls.

1. Controls may be deceased and/or living.
2. Controls may be randomly selected or matched to the cases.
3. Controls may be limited to persons with selected causes of death.

It seems logical to choose as controls only persons who are deceased, since the cases are deceased. However, this is not an absolute necessity. Also, it is a matter of preference whether matched or nonmatched controls are selected.

Matching is done in the selection of controls if it is desired to control potential confounding in the design of the study. Common matching factors include age, race, and sex. In order to increase the stability of any association with work history, two to four controls per case are usually selected. In a matched analyses, little further efficiency is gained with more than four controls per case.

Instead of selecting matched controls, one can simply select a random sample of noncases and evaluate possible confounding in the analysis. If this strategy is elected, it is frequently useful to select more than four controls per case, since if, for example, age turns out to be confounding, there may be some age strata with a high case:control ratio. Of course one has some idea as to the likelihood of confounding by age, since data on the age of the entire cohort are available prior to the selection of the controls.

In the selection of controls, it is always desirable to have some variability in the control diagnoses. If controls are selected from only one diagnostic category, interpretation of any association of work area with disease will be difficult. One will not know whether the cases were exposed too much or the controls too little. If there are several diagnostic categories among the controls, the percentage of persons with exposure to the many work areas are compared within the controls as well as between the cases and controls.

In analyzing matched data, it is useful to evaluate whether the matching was of any value. The easiest way to do this is compute the odds ratio on the matched data and on the data with the matching broken (See Chapter 4). If the matched and the unmatched odds ratios are essentially the same, a simple, unmatched analysis will suffice. This is especially useful if it is desired to control for factors not matched upon.

In assessing the association of work area with disease, similar strategies may be employed as in cohort studies. Each person may be categorized in each work area within which he worked, or he may be categorized only in his usual work area. Further, only persons who have worked some minimum number of years in a given work area may be considered.

The only reasons to do a case-control study within a cohort are time and money. There is no increase in scientific validity, since the information collected would be available if work histories for the entire cohort were reviewed. However, since the savings in time and money may be considerable, such studies have an important place in occupational epidemiology.

B. Example — Rubber Workers

At the same time the mortality study among B. F. Goodrich employees was being conducted, similar studies were being carried out in other rubber companies by the University of North Carolina School of Public Health. In one of these, excesses of lymphosarcoma (14 observed, 6.2 expected) and of leukemia (16 observed, 12.5 ex-

Table 6.21
DIFFERENCE BETWEEN CASES OF LYMPHATIC LEUKEMIA AND CONTROLS IN YEARS SPENT IN SELECTED DEPARTMENTAL GROUPINGS

Department group	Difference between cases and controls in years
Heavy solvent exposure	0.6
Medium solvent exposure	3.1
Light solvent exposure	3.6
Compounding and mixing	−0.2
Milling	−0.2
Extrusion	−0.2
Curing	−2.0
General service	−1.7
All other	−4.7

pected) were seen among a cohort of 6678 male hourly employees.[24] Because of the complexity of the personnel records for this cohort and because of changes in the departmental coding system from one era to another, it was judged prohibitively expensive to review the work records of the whole cohort.

Instead, a case-control study was conducted.[18] Cases were 88 persons with a lymphatic or hematopoietic disease (which includes leukemia and lymphosarcoma). Controls were decedents of other causes matched in a 4:1 ratio to cases on the basis of age, race, sex, and plant. The detailed work histories of the 88 cases and the 352 controls were reviewed.

The primary analysis focused on the number of years the cases and controls had spent in defined departments, i.e., the number of years of "exposure". As seen in Table 6.21, cases with lymphatic leukemia had spent more time in the departments with solvent exposure than had controls. By contrast, controls had spent more time in most of the other departmental groupings.

If information had been collected on the solvent exposure history for all 6678 workers, SMRs for lymphatic leukemia could have been computed for each solvent exposure grouping: high, medium, low, or none. However, the cost would have been greater. The association between lymphatic leukemia and solvent exposure in this study is similar to that reported among the B. F. Goodrich employees.[3]

REFERENCES

1. **Monson, R. R. and Nakano, K. K.,** Mortality among rubber workers. I. White male union employees in Akron, Ohio, *Am. J. Epidemiol.,* 103, 284, 1976.
2. **Monson, R. R. and Nakano, K. K.,** Mortality among rubber workers. II. Other employees, *Am. J. Epidemiol.,* 103, 297, 1976.
3. **Monson, R. R. and Fine, L. J.,** Cancer mortality and morbidity among rubber workers, *J. Nat. Cancer Inst.,* 61, 1047, 1978.
4. **Delzell, E. and Monson, R. R.,** Patterns of mortality among rubber workers, unpublished data.

5. **Stanislawczyk, K., Kaminski, R., and Spirtas, R.,** A Proportional Mortality Analysis of a Chemical Plant in Massachusetts, National Institute for Occupational Health and Safety, Washington, D.C., May, 1978.

6. **Killeen, J.,** A Proportional Mortality Study of Monsanto-Indian Orchard Employees, Monsanto Chemical Company, St. Louis, March, 1978.

7. **Najarian, T. and Colton, T.,** Mortality from leukemia and cancer in shipyard nuclear workers, *Lancet*, 1, 1018, 1978.

8. **Redmond, C.K., Smith, E. M., Lloyd, J. W., and Rush, H. W.,** Long-term mortality study of steelworkers. III. Follow-up, *J. Occup. Med.*, 11, 513, 1969.

9. **Boice, J. D., Jr.,** Follow-up methods to trace women treated for pulmonary tuberculosis, *Am. J. Epidemiol.*, 107, 127, 1978.

10. Eighth International Classification of Diseases, PHS Publ. No. 1693, U.S. Department of Health, Education and Welfare, Washington, D.C., 1967.

11. **Duck, B. W., Carter, J. T., and Coombes, E. J.,** Mortality study of workers in a polyvinyl-chloride production plant, *Lancet*, 2, 1197, 1975.

12. **Wagoner, J. K., Infante, P. F., and Saracci, R.,** Vinyl chloride and mortality?, *Lancet*, 2, 194, 1976.

13. **Rothman, K. J. and Monson, R. R.,** Survival in trigeminal neuralgia, *J. Chronic Dis.*, 26, 303, 1973.

14. **McMichael, A. J.,** Standardized mortality ratios and the "Healthy worker effect". Scratching beneath the surface, *J. Occup. Med.*, 18, 165, 1976.

15. **Fox, A. J. and Collier, P. F.,** Low mortality rates in industrial cohort studies due to selection of work and survival in the industry, *Br. J. Prev. Soc. Med.*, 30, 225, 1976.

16. **Monson, R. R.,** Analysis of relative survival and proportional mortality, *Comput. Biomed. Res.*, 7, 325, 1974.

17. **Gaffey, W. R.,** A critique of the standardized mortality ratio, *J. Occup. Med.*, 18, 157, 1976.

18. **McMichael, A. J., Spirtas, R., Kupper, L. L., and Gamble, J. F.,** Solvent exposure and leukemia among rubber workers, *J. Occup. Med.*, 17, 234, 1974.

19. **Infante, P. F., Rinsky, R. A., and Wagoner, J. F.,** Leukemia in benzene workers, *Lancet*, 2, 76, 1977.

20. **Kupper, L. L., McMichael, A. J., Symons, M. J., and Most, B. M.,** On the utility of proportional mortality analysis, *J. Chronic Dis.*, 31, 15, 1978.

21. **Creech, J. L., Jr. and Johnson, M. N.,** Angiosarcoma of liver in the manufacture of polyvinyl chloride, *J. Occup. Med.*, 16, 150, 1974.

22. **Monson, R. R., Peters, J. M., and Johnson, M. N.,** Proportional mortality among vinyl chloride workers, *Lancet*, 2, 397, 1974.

23. **Tabershaw, I. R. and Gaffey, W. R.,** Mortality study of workers in the manufacture of vinyl chloride and its polymers, *J. Occup. Med.*, 16, 509, 1974.

24. **McMichael, A. J., Spirtas, R., and Kupper, L. L.,** An epidemiologic study of mortality within a cohort of rubber workers, 1964—72, *J. Occup. Med.*, 16, 458, 1974.

Chapter 7
STUDIES OF MORBIDITY

I. INTRODUCTION

Whereas mortality studies essentially rely on data that are collected from a cohort of workers, morbidity studies may take several forms:

1. An acute outbreak of illness among a group of workers that is attributed to some toxic exposure usually takes the form of a case report from the clinical setting. The disease occurs shortly after exposure to some agent and no formal study is required. Such reports are analagous to acute outbreaks in infectious disease epidemiology.
2. Case-control studies are done in a hospital setting to evaluate previous exposures in persons with and without a specific disease. Occupational histories are obtained as part of the person's exposure history.
3. Cross-sectional surveys are done on a group of workers that relate current health status to current employment. The basic problem in interpretation of data from these surveys is to determine the time sequence between employment and some abnormal health outcome. One way to overcome this interpretative difficulty is to repeat the survey on the same workers. By so doing, the evaluation becomes a prospective cohort study.
4. Formal cohort studies, either retrospective or prospective, are done to assess the rates of many diseases in relation to some occupational exposure.

In mortality studies, death rates among some occupational group are frequently compared to the rates in some outside general population. Thus there is a basis of comparison, albeit imperfect, that can be used in different cohort studies. In morbidity studies, however, no comparison with outside data usually is possible. Some internal control must be built into the design of most morbidity studies. While this internal control is generally a desirable characteristic of all epidemiologic studies, it does not necessarily lead to unambiguous interpretation of the data. A difference in the disease rate between two groups may be the result of a rate that is too high in one group or too low in the second.

II. CASE REPORTS

A. MDA and Hepatitis

Between 1966 and 1972, 12 employees of an industrial plant developed hepatitis.[1] Initially, the disease was thought to be viral. However, after eight cases had occurred, it was recognized that all were employed in the same room of the plant; there were no cases elsewhere in the plant. Further, all men worked with methylenedianiline (MDA), which had been identified as causing an outbreak of hepatitis in 1965.[2]

In 1971, a formal retrospective investigation of this outbreak was begun.[1] This evaluation was analagous to that conducted in infectious disease epidemiology, for example, following a food poisoning epidemic. The persons who had had the disease were examined and their work characteristics were related to their hepatitis. Each had developed hepatitis within 1 to 4 weeks after initial exposure to MDA.

"Unfortunately, it had often happened in industry that the toxicity of a substance has been neither recognized nor accepted because not everyone exposed to it was af-

Table 7.1
CASE-CONTROL COMPARISON OF DBCP
WORKERS

	Sperm count	
	Low (n = 11)	Normal (n = 11)
Average age	32.7	26.7
Average years exposed to DBCP[a]	8.0	0.1

[a] $P < 0.01$.

fected.''[1] An attack rate less than 100% is also the rule in infectious disease epidemiology; everyone who eats the contaminated potato salad does not become ill. In spite of this incomplete occurrence of the disease, the rate ratio was infinity: the rate of hepatitis in the nonexposed worker during these years was zero. Thus even though this outbreak was evaluated in the clinical setting, unstated epidemiologic principles form the basis of data interpretation.

Outbreaks such as this should not simply be worked up and then forgotten. Even though the 12 workers recovered from their hepatitis, the possible long-term sequelae must be considered. These workers and other persons like them must be followed for many years to determine whether any other illness might occur, especially cancer. A clinical problem, once it has been resolved. must be continued as an epidemiologic problem. A report of a series of cases should become the start of a prospective cohort study. These 12 workers, together with exposed, nondiseased workers and with nonexposed workers should be kept track of for the indefinite future.

B. Dioxin and Chloracne

Chloracne, a severe form of acne, is recognized as being the result of exposure to chlorinated aromatic compounds.[3] Thus persons who work with these compounds must be carefully monitored for the development of chloracne.

In 1970, three laboratory scientists were working with dioxin under controlled laboratory conditions. Two of the three developed typical chloracne; the third did not.[4] Three years later one of the persons who had chloracne and the third person developed vague systemic symptoms: headache, fatigue, indigestion, excess hair growth. All three had serum cholesterol levels above 300 mg/100 ml.

Whether these general symptoms represent a delayed result of the exposure to dioxin is unknown. However, these symptoms underscore the need for continued follow-up of persons who experience an acute illness due to an industrial exposure.

C. DBCP and Infertility

The two outbreaks described above were of overt illness that could be related to an industrial exposure. However, industrial exposures may also lead to physiologic abnormalities that may go undetected for several years. Men working with a nematocide, 1,2-dibromo-3-chloropropane (DBCP) recognized among themselves that few had recently fathered children.[5] On investigation, 11 men were found to have very low sperm counts.

After recognition of this "outbreak" of infertility, a case-control comparison was made among all workers with DBCP (Table 7.1). The cases, those with low sperm counts, were older and had worked many more years with DBCP than had the controls.

In interpreting the data in Table 7.1, several points must be considered. Clearly the cases are older than the controls. Whether this difference is statistically significant or not is irrelevant. Even if the cases were aged 26.8 years on the average, they would be older than the controls. What is relevant is whether sperm count varies with age, and if so to what extent, so that control for confounding due to age is necessary. While sperm count indeed decreases with age, all men aged 30 to 40 or so are not infertile. Thus on judgment alone one can decide that age need not be controlled in this comparison.

The fact that the difference in average years of exposure of DBCP is statistically significant at the 0.01 level indicates that the data are stable. The p-value of course does not indicate that DBCP caused the infertility. That connection again is a matter of judgment. There may be other chemicals to which the men with infertility were exposed.

D. Comment

The initial recognition of the above episode by the persons affected points out a valuable source of information on industrial health — the worker.[6] In any epidemiologic surveillance system within industry, worker access is essential. Frequently, potential adverse health effects can be recognized at the time of initial exposure and corrective action taken.

Medical records maintained by industrial organizations, also, frequently contain information that can be used by the epidemiologist. The primary purpose of the medical record is to keep a record of the clinical aspects of a person's health status. As such, a description may be made of acute illnesses that may have an industrial component to their etiology. The potential long-term sequelae of such illnesses are not readily recognized by the clinician. However, just as persons with chloracne may have delayed symptoms, so may persons with other industrially-induced skin disease be subject to some more serious chronic disease. Medical records form a potential valuable source of information that can be used for retrospective cohort studies of persons who have had minor illnesses because of work-related exposures.

III. CASE-CONTROL STUDIES

A. Study Rationale

Whereas cohort studies are typically done to evaluate the effects of some exposure, case-control studies are done to assess exposures that are associated with some disease. For this reason, cohort studies are more naturally suited to the evaluation of health patterns among some (exposed) occupational group.

However, case-control studies have an important place in the preliminary assessment of the association between occupation and disease. In case-control studies, persons with specific diseases can be asked about their complete occupational history. In so doing, information on a broad spectrum of occupational exposures can be obtained. By contrast, in a cohort study of an occupational group, information on occupation is heavily concentrated on the exposures of one industry.

The price paid for the potential breadth of occupational information in case-control studies is imprecise measurement of occupational exposures and small numbers of diseased persons with specific occupations. Information on occupation is typically obtained through personal interviews and rarely is documented further. Unless the study is conducted in an area with a predominant industry, tens or hundreds of occupations may be included. As a result, any associations between disease and occupation that are detected tend to be unstable.

B. Procedure

1. Collection of Data

Case-control studies typically are done in hospital settings. An investigator is interested in a disease and wishes to obtain information on the possible precursors of that disease. He makes arrangements with one or more hospitals to collect data from persons with that disease and from controls.

a. Selection of Cases

An initial consideration is whether to study incident cases or prevalent cases. Incident cases are persons newly diagnosed with the disease of interest. Prevalent cases are persons who have been diagnosed in the past. One can assemble a group of prevalent cases faster inasmuch as they occurred over some period in the past. To assemble a group of incident cases, the investigator must age along with the unspecified study population as in a prospective cohort study.

It is generally considered best to conduct case-control studies on incident cases. Such persons are seen early in their disease and thus are closer in time to any antecedent exposures. The effects of the disease may not have affected the person's ability or inclination to recall past information. Further, a series of prevalent cases is usually made up of persons with different characteristics of survival. Persons with rapidly fatal disease will tend to be underrepresented in a series of prevalent cases.

b. Selection of Controls

The selection of a series of control patients is the most important aspect of a case-control study. Ideally, the controls should be representative of the population from which the cases derived, so that the occupational histories of the controls can form a basis of comparison for those of the controls. However, usually in hospital-based studies, the cases come from no defined population. To the extent that there is selective admission of persons with specific diseases and specific occupations, case-control comparability may be difficult to assess.

With respect to hospital controls, it is desirable that there be a spectrum of diagnoses, so that the distribution of occupations within the controls can be assessed. If some occupation is more common among one disease group than among a second, it is uncertain as to which percentage is abnormal. However, if among ten disease groups, only one has a high proportion of persons with some occupation, it is more likely that the high proportion is atypical.

In the selection of hospital controls, persons with diseases that have a recognized occupational component should not be included. For example, if one is assessing the association between heart disease and hard rock mining, persons with silicosis or with emphysema would not comprise a logical control group. Many of the persons with these diagnoses have an occupational disease, and the prevalence of hard rock miners would be high. The control group in this example is clearly not representative of the general population from which the cases came.

The decision as to which disease groups to include among the controls is clearly judgmental and subject to differences of opinion. Perhaps the best strategy is to include marginal groups in the collection of the data and to consider excluding them from the analysis. By so doing data are available that can be used in deciding whether or not to exclude a specific group.

Controls also can be selected from the general population. By so doing, one is comparing the occupational histories of a diseased group to those of a group that is essentially healthy. Fewer questions can be raised as to the possible biased occupational patterns among controls who have other diseases. Further, if the case group is population-based, that is, if all the incident cases in some defined population over some time period are included, the use of population controls means that the data are similar to cohort data. The controls are a specified sample of all of the noncases in the population, and inferences can readily be made to the entire population.

The advantages of population controls are not absolute, however. Clearly, it costs more to identify and interview controls at home rather than in the hospital. Further, if there is selective admission of diseased persons to the hospital, and if the selection is related to occupation, hospital controls may be more appropriate than population controls.

c. Collection of Study Data

Information on a person's occupational history and on other exposure data are typically obtained by questionnaire — either self-administered or by interview. There may be three levels in the collection of a person's occupational history. If the study is exploratory, the patient simply relates in chronologic order his lifetime occupations, giving the years each occupation started and stopped. Each occupation should be characterized as to nature of the work done and the company of employment. A second level of questions may be asked, in which the patient is asked about general exposures such as dusts, fumes, radiation, noise, etc. Finally, the patient may be asked about exposure to specific substances, such as benzene, cadmium, silica dust, etc.

The decision as to how detailed an occupational history to get depends upon the reason for the study. If questions on occupation are included only as part of a general survey of exposure, a fairly brief occupational history is all that is realistic. In the absence of specific questions that are being addressed, it is not worth the expense to spend an hour per patient getting detailed occupation histories. However, if one of the primary reasons for the study is to assess the relationship between a specific disease and a specific substance, a detailed occupational history with respect to that substance is needed.

Case-control studies are subject to observation bias in the collection of the information on occupation. If the patients or the interviewers are aware of some specific disease-occupation association that is being evaluated, it clearly is possible that persons with the disease will report their occupational history in a manner different from the controls. It is important that in the collection of data in a case-control study, data be collected in a similar manner from cases and controls. The reason for the study must be presented to each group as a general survey of health and illness rather than as a specific survey of a disease and an occupation.

2. Analysis of Data

In Chapter 4 the basic analysis of case-control data is described. For most case-control studies, meaningful rates of disease cannot be computed since the ratio of cases to controls may be set by the investigator. Even if all persons in a hospital group are included in the study, the percentage (rate) of persons with, say lung cancer, is not the same as the percentage in the general population.

In a cohort study, the measure of association between exposure and disease is the rate ratio. By analogy, one might expect that in a case-control study an epidemiologist might compute an "exposure ratio" — the ratio of the exposure percentage in the cases to that in the controls. While there is no scientific reason not to use this measure, the odds ratio has become the usual measure of association in a case-control study. Since the basic motivation in epidemiology is to determine factors that influence the rate of disease in a population, the rate ratio is viewed as the best measure of association. The odds ratio is a better approximation of the rate ratio than is the exposure ratio.

The next step is to attempt to uncover confounding factors that may have accounted for any association seen. (If the odds ratio is 1.0, negative confounding could be searched for, although this is rarely a useful exercise.) The easiest way to search for confounding is to cross-tabulate each potential confounding factor with the disease and/or with the exposure. The only factors that can be confounding are those that are related to both exposure and disease.

Confounding may be controlled in a variety of ways (see Chapter 4):

1. Cases and controls may be separated into strata of the confounding factor, so that there is no association between disease and the factor in each stratum. A Mantel-Haenszel standardized odds ratio is then computed.[7]
2. Matching in the analysis may be done for the factor(s) that is (are) confounding. For each case, one or more controls are selected from the pool of controls. A standardized odds ratio is computed on the basis of a matched analysis.
3. A multivariate analysis may be done. As many factors as desired are entered into a model along with information on exposure for cases and controls. A standardized odds ratio is computed.

My preference is to stratify. Usually, many factors can be shown not to be confounding simply because they are not associated with exposure or with disease. Control for 2 to 5 factors by simultaneous stratification is usually possible. Stratification is straight-forward, understandable, and inexpensive.

I prefer not to do matched analyses. While it is not difficult nor expensive to select matched controls from the pool of controls, it may be difficult to match each case exactly to one or more control. Also, in a matched analysis all of the data at hand is usually not used, and the stability of the standardized odds ratio may be less than that computed through stratification. However, other epidemiologists do prefer matched analyses, and there is no theoretical reason not to do them.

In the analysis of case-control data, multivariate techniques are becoming more widely used. It is appealing to be able to enter data on all variables into a model and not have to limit the scope of the analysis. However, before multivariate techniques supplant the simpler and more traditional methods, more experience is needed in the comparison of the analysis of the same data using different techniques. Multivariate techniques tend to be opaque to the consumer; it is difficult to grasp the machinations through which the data go in a multivariate analysis. Further, certain theoretical statistical assumptions, e.g., normally distributed continuous data, tend to be violated by many epidemiologic data. In spite of this, as the results of multivariate analyses accord with the results of simple analyses and with common sense, these methods will become more widely used and understood.

Having controlled for confounding, one presents the standardized odds ratios. A measure of stability may be computed so as to indicate whether or not the odds ratio is a stable estimate.

As in cohort studies, the basic nature of occupational data complicates the analysis of case-control studies. Many people have had a variety of occupations and a variety of exposures. There likely is interdependence between several occupations and the separation of the effects of each of the occupations may be difficult.

Three different strategies are useful in defining occupation (1) a person can be counted only in his usual occupation; (2) a person can be counted in each of his occupations; and (3) a person can be counted in each of his occupations, but strata can be constructed according to number of years worked.

In strategy one, the simplest presentation of the data is to display the percentages of usual occupations among the various case and control disease groups. The odds ratio can be used as the measure of association. If control is to be done for the effects of confounding factors, the Mantel-Haenszel odds ratio is computed.[7]

In strategy two, all of the information on occupation and disease can be used. However, there is a tendency toward the dilution of any association because of the inclusion of persons who worked in an occupation for a short period of time. Also, if two or more occupations are interrelated, it may not be clear which occupation is important in any association.

Strategy three appears to be a compromise between the other two strategies: occupations of short duration can be excluded, but a more comprehensive use of the data is possible.

If an association is found between occupation and disease, and if that association is based on stable numbers of persons, latency analysis may be done.[8] It is of interest to describe differences between cases and controls with respect to number of years worked in the suspect occupation, age, and year started working, and number of years between start of work and diagnosis of disease (latency). While these analyses are analagous to those conducted on cohort data, interpretation of the results is conceptually more difficult. The cases do not derive from a defined cohort, and the latent period is to some extent a reflection of the distribution of the age at diagnosis. Ideally, associations seen in case-control data should be evaluated further in cohort data.

C. Example — Bladder Cancer
1. A Population-Based Study with Controls from the General Population

Between 1/1/67 and 6/30/68 all newly diagnosed (incident) cases of bladder cancer in the Greater Boston area were identified.[8-10] These cases were identified by a periodic search of pathology logs at 111 hospitals. Controls were selected at random from a roster prepared from annual Massachusetts Resident's Lists. The age and resident distribution of persons in the roster roughly conformed to that of the cases. (See also Chapter 3.)

Interviews were conducted with both cases and controls at home. Information was obtained on smoking and drinking histories, and a life-time occupation history was taken. Open-ended questions were asked about the employing organization, the person's position, the age started and the years worked in each position, the specific duties performed and exposure to a variety of general substances (chemical, solutions, dusts, fumes, radiation).

Various analytic methods were used. Because this was a population-based study, incidence rates of bladder cancer could be computed as in a cohort study. This was done in the analysis of cigarette smoking.[10] In the analysis of occupational data, the observed number of cases with specified occupations were compared to the number expected if the cases had the same age and smoking distributions as the controls.[9] In the analysis of latency and other time variables, Mantel-Haenszel odds ratios were computed.[7,8]

In Tables 7.2 and 7.3 data are presented on the occupational patterns of the cases. In Table 7.2, a person is counted in each of his occupations; in Table 7.3 he is counted only once — in his usual occupation. The specific occupational categories are those which on a priori grounds were considered likely to be associated with bladder cancer. As seen in Table 7.2, a moderate association of bladder cancer was seen with the dyestuff, rubber, and leather occupational categories; the associations are based on reasonably large numbers. In Table 7.3, moderate associations are also seen for rubber and leather; however, no man with bladder cancer had spent his usual occupational life in

Table 7.2
OBSERVED AND EXPECTED NUMBER OF PERSONS WITH BLADDER CANCER IN BOSTON WHO EVER WORKED IN AN OCCUPATION CATEGORY

Occupation category	Bladder cancer cases		Odds
	Observed	Expected[a]	ratio[b]
Dyestuff	7	3.9	2.2
Rubber	51	36.8	1.6
Leather	79	41.5	2.0
Printing	15	16.1	1.1
Paint	28	22.7	1.2
Petroleum	102	102.4	1.0
Other organic chemicals	14	10.9	1.4
Other chemicals	18	20.9	1.0
Other occupation	927	985.8	1.0

[a]   Case occupations expected on the basis of the control distribution.
[b]   Relative to a ratio of 1.0 for "other occupation", controlled for age and cigarette smoking.

Table 7.3
OBSERVED AND EXPECTED NUMBER OF PERSONS WITH BLADDER CANCER IN BOSTON WHO USUALLY WORKED IN AN OCCUPATION CATEGORY[a]

Occupation category	Bladder cancer cases		Odds
	Observed	Expected	ratio
Dyestuffs	0	1.8	0
Rubber	19	11.6	1.7
Leather	21	12.1	1.7
Printing	5	7.7	0.8
Paint	11	8.7	1.3
Petroleum	34	34.4	1.1
Other organic chemicals	3	2.0	1.6
Other chemicals	6	6.9	0.9
Other occupations	246	259.8	1.0

[a]   See footnotes to Table 7.2.

the dyestuffs industry. For the other suspect occupations, there was little indication of an association with bladder cancer.

The numbers of the specific occupations listed in these Tables is a reflection of the occupational pattern of workers in the Boston area, not of the pattern of persons with bladder cancer. The absence of any occupation from the listing does not mean that it is not a cause of bladder cancer, but only that it is not a common occupation in the Boston area.

On the basis of the data in Table 7.2, the dyestuffs, rubber, and leather occupations were classified as hazardous, since data consistent with the *a priori* judgement of hazard were obtained in this study. In Table 7.4, the age at initial employment in a hazardous occupation was compared between cases and controls. A strong association is

Table 7.4

NUMBER OF PERSONS WITH
BLADDER CANCER IN
BOSTON AND CONTROLS
ACCORDING TO AGE AT
INITIAL EMPLOYMENT IN A
HAZARDOUS OCCUPATION[a]

Age at employment (yr)	Cases	Controls	Odds ratios
12—15	26	10	4.8
16—20	57	30	2.5
21—25	22	16	2.0
26—35	11	14	1.1
≥36	14	17	1.3
Never	217	277	1.0

[a] Dyestuffs, rubber or leather.

Table 7.5

NUMBER OF PERSONS
WITH BLADDER CANCER
IN BOSTON AND
CONTROLS ACCORDING
TO NUMBER OF YEARS
BETWEEN FIRST
EMPLOYMENT IN A
HAZARDOUS OCCUPATION[a]
AND DIAGNOSIS
(LATENCY)

Latency (yrs)	Cases	Controls	Odds ratio
≤30	11	8	1.8
31—40	19	10	2.4
41—50	39	13	3.8
≥51	36	25	1.8

[a] Dyestuffs, rubber, leather.

seen in that cases were over-represented by an early age at employment. In Table 7.5, the strongest association with latency is at 41 to 50 years.

The interpretation of these data on bladder cancer and occupation must take into account other data. The excess number of cases with prior employment in the dyestuffs, rubber, and leather industries argues for a causal association, in that similar excesses had been seen earlier. The data on age at starting and latency, however, have not been replicated. Further, the specific substances that may be responsible for the excess cases of bladder cancer are unknown. In the case-control setting on occupation, it is difficult to do more than point the need for follow-up studies in specific occupational groups.

2. A Population-Based Study with Hospital Controls

Between 1959 and 1967, all newly diagnosed persons at two hospitals in Leeds, England, were asked about their occupational histories.[11] Inasmuch as these hospitals served a defined population, the case series may be thought of as population-based. Incidence rates of bladder cancer according to the various population characteristics could be computed.

The control series was not selected at the same time as the persons with bladder cancer. Rather, the controls were selected from controls who had been interviewed in a previous study of lung cancer between 1955 and 1958; they were surgical patients who did not have cancer. For each case, a control was selected and matched on sex, age, residence, and smoking habit.

The analysis was a matched-pairs analysis. If both the case and control had a specific occupation or if neither had the occupation, they were not counted. The data as to usual occupation are presented in Table 7.6.

As can be seen, the occupational distribution is quite different from that in Boston. There were very few dye or rubber workers, so that no assessment could be made of the role of these occupations in bladder cancer. Among leather workers, however, the

Table 7.6
NUMBER OF PERSONS WITH
BLADDER CANCER IN LEEDS AND
CONTROLS ACCORDING TO USUAL
OCCUPATION

Occupation category	Cases	Controls	Odds ratio[a]
Farmers, etc.	15	14	1.1
Miners	29	22	1.3
Gas, coke, chemical	6	4	1.5
Glass and ceramic	3	5	0.6
Forge and foundry	7	9	0.8
Electric	9	6	1.5
Engineers	61	51	1.2
Wood	8	11	0.7
Leather	0	7	0
Textiles	20	11	1.9
Clothing	19	11	1.8
Food	9	5	1.8
Paper	2	7	0.3
All other	152	177	0.9
Total	340	340	

[a] Odds ratio = number of cases ÷ number of controls.

odds ratio was 0.0: no cases and seven controls had their usual employment in the leather industry.

3. A Hospital-Based Study with Hospital Controls

Between 1969 and 1974, persons with bladder cancer in 17 hospitals in six U.S. cities were interviewed.[12] As part of the interview, information on occupation was obtained. Controls were a 1:1 group matched on sex, race, hospital, and age. Although this was a matched case-control study, an unmatched analysis was done. With respect to occupational history, this probably has little effect inasmuch as there is little concordance of occupations. The data are presented in Table 7.7. Again, the occupational groupings are general and the number of persons in each category is small. No strong associations are seen, even though these occupations were suspected *a priori* as being associated with bladder cancer.

D. Comment

As the data in these tables suggest, case-control studies are of a limited usage in occupational epidemiology. The data must be obtained by interview and usually cannot be documented. Little specific detail as to exposure can be obtained. The occupations that can be evaluated are restricted to those present in the particular geographic area. The number of persons in any one occupational group is small.

As will be described in Chapter 8, on-going case-control surveillance for associations between drugs and diseases has been found to be useful. The adaptation of this methodology to evaluate associations with occupations may prove useful. It is essential, however, to target the surveillance system so that specific associations can be studied. Such a surveillance system may prove of value more in the measuring of known occupational-disease associations than in the identification of new associations.

Table 7.7
NUMBER OF PERSONS WITH BLADDER CANCER IN THE U.S. AND CONTROLS ACCORDING TO WHETHER A PERSON EVER WORKED IN THE OCCUPATION CATEGORY

Occupation category	Cases	Controls
Rubber	3	1
Paint	10	13
Dye	7	7
Chemicals	13	11
Textile	14	10
Dust	24	19
Metal	54	64
Grease and oil	10	7

IV. CROSS-SECTIONAL STUDIES

A. Study Rationale

Frequently in occupational settings a survey is made of disease prevalence in active workers. Such surveys are not cohort studies, for workers are not followed up to measure new cases of illness. Also, these surveys are not case-control studies, for persons with and without disease are not selected and asked about past occupational exposures. Data from prevalence surveys are cross-sectional; selection of the study population is done without regard to exposure or disease status. The basic difficulty in cross-sectional data is in interpretation; did the exposure lead to the disease or did persons with certain medical conditions select specific jobs?

Cross-sectional studies are useful to assess whether associations exist between exposure and disease. If associations are found, more definitive studies can be done to assess the association. In particular, two cross-sectional studies done on the same population at different points in time are quite similar to prospective cohort studies.

B. Procedure

In cross-sectional studies, data are collected on exposure and disease at the same time. Current occupation is assessed in terms of level of exposure to some job or some substance. Current health status is measured as either a present/absent condition or on some continuous scale. Correlations may be made between two sets of continuous data, or the data can be degraded into a 2 × 2 table. Discrete data can be analyzed as a 2 × 2 or some larger contingency table. The procedures for the collection and analysis of data are to some extent similar to those used for case-control studies.

However, there are obvious differences. The data are collected in the industrial setting rather than in the hospital. Information on exposure can frequently be obtained directly from records or from industrial hygiene measurements. Information on disease tends to be measurements of physiologic abnormalities rather than of overt illness.

In the collection of data on exposure on an individual, precise measurements usually are not possible. Thus data on dose are only an approximation. This must be kept in mind in evaluating dose-response relationships. Because of random misclassification of exposure, any true dose-exposure relationship may be softened. However, in case-control studies, it rarely is feasible even to attempt an evaluation of dose-response relationships.

Table 7.8
DESCRIPTIVE DATA ON TWO GROUPS OF
RUBBER WORKERS

Variable	Curing workers	Controls
No. of men	121	189
Average age, year	40.3	39.0
Average height, cm	178.6	175.4
Average years employed, year	16.0	13.9
Current smoker, %	47.9	44.4

C. Example — Respiratory Disease

1. Rubber Workers

A cross-sectional study of respiratory disease was done among curing workers in the rubber industry.[13,14] During the curing of tires, workers are exposed to a fume containing a variety of potentially harmful substances. As controls, workers from a variety of jobs within the same plant were selected. Control workers were matched on age and duration of employment.

A standardized respiratory disease questionnaire was administered to each subject. Also, pulmonary function tests were administered twice at a 1-year interval. A basic measure of pulmonary function is the volume of air that can be exhaled in 1 sec, the forced expiratory volume ($FEV_{1.0}$).

As seen in Table 7.8, the group of curing workers were similar to the controls; there are more controls than exposed workers because the controls for several groups of exposed workers were combined. More curing workers than controls were current smokers, even though the excess was small. Since smoking is strongly associated with respiratory symptoms and with pulmonary function, it was decided to control for smoking.

Baseline cross-sectional data are presented in Table 7.9. Curing workers in general reported a higher prevalence or current history of a variety of respiratory symptoms. Their $FEV_{1.0}$, was similar to that of the controls. However, the residual $FEV_{1.0}$ was negative for the curing workers and positive for the controls. The residual $FEV_{1.0}$ is a standardized measure of pulmonary function that took into account age, height, and cigarette smoking.

It appears from the data in Table 7.9 that curing workers have had more respiratory disease than the controls. However, these data could arise either if persons with respiratory disease became curing workers or if exposure to the curing fume caused respiratory disease.

The 1 year change in $FEV_{1.0}$ is presented in Table 7.10. In most working populations, there is a 20 to 40 ml/year decrease in the $FEV_{1.0}$.[14] Thus the loss in the controls is slightly greater than that expected. However, among those curing workers who had worked for more than 10 years, the loss was substantially greater. This provides firmer evidence that working in the curing atmosphere had an effect on the lung.

2. Firefighters

During the period 1970—72 Boston firefighters were evaluated for the prevalence of chronic nonspecific respiratory disease (CNSRD). Questionnaire data on respiratory symptoms and pulmonary function tests were used to categorize each firefighter as to CNSRD. Specifically, CNSRD was defined as the presence of chronic nonproductive cough, chronic bronchitis, asthma, or chronic obstructive lung disease.

The data in Table 7.11 present the association of CNSRD according to smoking

Table 7.9

PERCENTAGE OF RUBBER WORKERS WITH RESPIRATORY SYMPTOMS AND BASELINE FEV$_{1.0}^{a}$

Symptom	Curing workers	Controls
Cough, 3 month	19.2	7.4
History of bronchitis	10.7	7.4
Wheezing	8.3	5.3
FEV$_{1.0}$, $_m l$	3731	3732
Residual	−74	27
FEV$_{1.0}$, $_m l$		

^{a} One second forced expiratory volume.

habits and years as a firefighter in men under the age of 35. The age distributions of the two groups of firefighters were similar. A strong association of CNSRD with smoking is apparent in each length of service group. Also, within each smoking stratum, men who worked as firefighters more than 0.5 years had higher rates of CNSRD than their newly employed co-workers. The rate ratio is higher in nonsmokers, suggesting that firefighting has more of an impact on the lungs of nonsmokers. Further, if the rate difference is computed (rate in 0.5 to 14 workers minus rate in <0.5 workers), a decreasing trend is seen with increasing smoking.

While these data are consistent with a chronic effect of firefighting on the lung, they are cross-sectional data. More definite evidence would come from a longitudinal evaluation of changes in CNSRD prevalence or in pulmonary function.

The prevalence survey was repeated in one year.[16] The change in FEV$_{1.0}$ during this year was related to the number of fires fought during that year (Table 7.12). A dose-response relationship between number of fires and loss in pulmonary function was observed.

D. Comment

Cross-sectional data similar to those discussed above will be forthcoming from the epidemiologic surveillance systems that are being set up in industry. As can be seen, the interpretation of these data is subject to ambiguity. However, the collection of cross-sectional data will be repeated periodically. The data then become longitudinal. The difference between two prevalence rates divided by the length of time between the two measurements is the incidence rate. It is likely that the comparison of these incidence rates among groups of workers will provide the most definitive evaluation of the effect of the industrial environment on health.

V. COHORT STUDIES

A. Study Rationale

In the discussion of cross-sectional data, it was emphasized that longitudinal data are more readily interpreted than cross-sectional data. Further, in industrial settings, the follow-up of a group of employed persons to measure rates of disease is more rational than the interview as to past occupation of a group of persons with disease. For these reasons, cohort studies are used in the evaluation of the mortality of employed populations.

Table 7.10

ONE-YEAR CHANGE IN $FEV_{1.0}$
ACCORDING TO DURATION OF
EXPOSURE

	Curing workers		Controls	
	<10 year	>10 year	<10 year	>10 year
$\Delta FEV_{1.0, ml}$	+11	−173	−73	−41

Table 7.11

PREVALENCE RATES OF CHRONIC
NONSPECIFIC RESPIRATORY DISEASE
(CNSRD) AMONG BOSTON FIREFIGHTERS
ACCORDING TO CIGARETTE USAGE AND
YEARS AS A FIREFIGHTER

Cigarettes smoked per day	Number of firefighters	Years as firefighters		Rate ratio
		<0.5	0.5—14	
0—14	193	3.6	11.6	3.2
15—24	120	15.0	21.3	1.4
≥25	100	31.5	35.9	1.1

Table 7.12

DECREMENT IN ONE
SECOND FORCED
EXPIRATORY VOLUME
($FEV_{1.0}$) ACCORDING TO
NUMBER OF FIRES
FOUGHT

Number of fires	Number of men	Decrement in $FEV_{1.0}$ (ml)
1—40	861	−49
41—99	216	−71
≥100	275	−109

Cohort studies also are of value in assessing morbidity. In particular, a prospective cohort study may be designed to evaluate the short-term effects of some exposure. The exposed and nonexposed populations can be characterized with relative precision, and all can be followed to measure the occurrence of new illness. Less complete data on individuals are available in retrospective cohort studies, which are conducted primarily to utilize information available from many years in the past.

B. Procedure

The basic procedures for retrospective cohort study on morbidity are similar to those for a study on mortality (Chapter 6). However, there are two important differences (1) illness cannot be reliably ascertained from the death certificate, and (2) internal rather than external comparisons of morbidity rates are necessary.

As discussed under cross-sectional studies, incident cases of disease can be ascertained if prevalence surveys are repeated periodically. While such surveys have the potential to measure the occurrence of illness with accuracy, they are expensive and time-consuming. Data that are collected for other purposes would be more comprehensive and less expensive. Examples include data from health insurance systems, from sickness and absence records, and from disability records. Historically, the basic problem with these records is that the diagnoses entered on these records are fairly nonspecific.

There are no national or regional morbidity rates that can be utilized in the manner of mortality rates. Data on incidence and prevalence of illness are collected by the National Health Survey (NHS).[17] However, the methods of data collection and the criteria for diagnosis used by the NHS differ from those used in industry. Because of this general noncomparability, routine comparisons between NHS data and data from industry are not possible. However, these data do form a useful basis of comparison to be included in any internal evaluation of rates.[18]

C. Examples

1. Morbidity Among Petroleum Refinery Workers

In 1973, cause-specific morbidity rates were measured in six petroleum refineries.[19] The basic study population was the mid-year number of employees at each refinery. Morbidity was assessed from medical absence records maintained by each refinery.

Age-adjusted cause-specific incidence rates of absence by cause are presented in Table 7.13 for three of the refineries. Interpretation of these data clearly is difficult. The fact that the overall rate in plant 4 is four times that in plant 3 does not necessarily mean that plant 4 is more dangerous. It may only mean that the record keeping system or the methods used to assess absence differ between the two plants.

This study was done to evaluate the feasibility of collecting data on morbidity within industry as a first step in the development of health and sickness monitoring systems. The study pointed out the need for three principles to be followed in the establishment of such systems:

1. The collection of data on morbidity should follow some defined protocol.
2. The measurement of exposure should be codified.
3. The measurement of disease should be codified.

The difference in disease rates among the refineries probably largely reflects different procedures in the collection and maintenance of health absence records. The use of refinery-wide rates was not likely to point out any excess rates of illness. Rather, within each refinery, rates of illness should be compared between specific jobs or specific exposures. The use of broad categories of disease tended to dampen any true association between work and disease. If work-related illness does occur, it is likely to be rather specific.

This study was the beginning of the on-going monitoring of morbidity within petroleum refineries. As such, it was a valuable link between ad hoc studies done to evaluate suspected dangers in industry and continuing epidemiologic surveillance systems. The lessons learned form the basis of more elaborate methods to assess the association between the work environment and employee health.

Table 7.13
AGE-ADJUSTED INCIDENCE
RATES[a] OF MEDICAL ABSENCE
BY CAUSE IN THREE OIL
REFINERIES

	Refinery number		
Cause	3	4	6
All malignancies	0	0.8	0
Lymphomas	0	0	0
Benign neoplasms	0.3	0.3	1.7
Circulatory disease	1.9	4.0	1.7
Respiratory disease	1.7	23.6	7.0
Digestive disease	2.7	4.2	8.4
Hernia	1.4	0.9	7.3
Genito-urinary disease	0.3	1.4	0
Skin disease	0.5	1.0	0
Infectious disease	0.3	12.5	0
Musculo-skeletal disease	1.4	4.7	3.3
Fractures, etc.	1.4	6.5	5.2
Other injuries	2.9	4.2	5.2
Other and unknown causes	3.7	9.6	3.5
All causes	17.1	72.8	36.1

[a]   Cases/100 men/year.

2. Respiratory Disability Among Rubber Workers

In addition to retrospective cohort studies of mortality among rubber workers, retrospective studies of morbidity have been done.[20] In this study, disease was measured as retirement due to pulmonary disability. No comparable population data exist for this disease.

Rather than analyzing rates of pulmonary disability according to exposure, a case-control evaluation was done within the cohort (see Chapter 6). Two control groups were selected and matched to the cases: one group was comprised of persons who retired because of other disabilities; the second contained nondisabled workers or retirees. Each group was matched to the cases on age, race, and sex.

The basic measure of exposure was the relative duration of service each worker had spent in specific work areas or exposed to general or specific substances. As seen in Table 7.14, there was no association between illness and the various exposure types or agents. However, persons who had retired because of pulmonary disability had spent a greater proportion of their working life in the curing preparation and curing work areas. These data are consistent with those found in another rubber plant.[13,14]

In this situation, a case-control analysis of cohort data was quite useful. It was necessary to collect work history information on only 365 workers rather than on the 4302 workers in the cohort. Clearly, this approach was less expensive. Had the work history data already been available on all members of the cohort, analysis could have been done of the incidence rate of pulmonary disability among the various exposure groups.

3. Cancer Morbidity Among Rubber Workers

In Chapter 6, results of mortality study among rubber workers were presented. In an extension of that study, morbidity from cancer was assessed.[21]

Table 7.14
DURATION OF SERVICE (YEARS/100 PERSON-
YEARS EXPOSURE) IN RUBBER INDUSTRY WORK
AREAS

Exposure	Pulmonary disabled retirement (n = 73)	Disabled controls (n = 146)	Nondisabled controls (n = 146)
Types			
Dust	22.4	19.4	22.2
Fumes	18.7	18.6	20.6
Vapors	30.9	30.7	32.0
Work areas			
Mixing	5.6	4.6	5.1
Milling	2.0	5.5	7.3
Curing preparation	7.2	1.1	0.8
Curing	9.1	6.3	4.5
Agents			
Talc	20.2	22.8	26.1
Carbon black	7.6	10.0	12.4

Newly diagnosed cases of cancer were identified through the tumor registries maintained by four Akron-area hospitals. The names of these persons were compared to the names of B. F. Goodrich rubber workers. Clearly, this procedure did not identify all cases of cancer among the cohort of rubber workers. Therefore, no comparison could be made with any external source of data on cancer morbidity.

However, it was assumed that the under-ascertainment of cancer was not related to the work area within the plant. While this assumption could not be tested, the four hospitals surveyed represent most of the medical-care facilities within the Akron area. Thus, even though persons from different work areas may go to different hospitals for the identification and treatment of their cancer, they should have been included in the survey.

Cancer morbidity rates were computed according to work area. The rates for work areas with high rates were compared to the rates for work areas with low rates. This procedure clearly is a matter of inspection of the data. Interpretation must rely on comparison with data from other sources. For each cancer, some work areas have higher rates simply because of chance.

Data on selected types of cancer are presented in Table 7.15. The excess lung cancer among curing workers is consistent with the excess pulmonary morbidity among curing workers.[13,14,20] A causal interpretation of the association is a distinct possibility. Certainly it is prudent to act as if the association is causal and to reduce exposure to the curing fume.

Whether the excesses in the other two work areas represent causal associations is unknown. The data on lung cancer among workers with tire molds are unstable (small number of cases, high standard error). The data on fuel cells/deicers are unusual in that persons with relatively short exposure have a higher rate of lung cancer than those with longer exposure. This inverse dose-response relationship might be taken as evidence against a causal interpretation. However, the measurement of years worked in specific work areas was imprecise; the difference in the two fuel cell/deicer rates could simply be due to chance.

Table 7.15
MORBIDITY RATES OF SELECTED CANCER
AMONG RUBBER WORKERS ACCORDING TO
WORK AREA

Type of cancer	Work area and minimum years in area[a]	Total cases	Standardized rate[b]	Rate ratio
Lung	Tire curing, 5 +	31	150(27)	2.2
	Tire molds, 5 +	10	136(43)	2.0
	Fuel cells/deicers, 5 +	26	97(20)	1.4
	Fuel cells/deicers, 0—4	20	134(34)	1.9
	Residual	196	69(5)	1.0
Skin	Tire assembly, 5 +	12	47(14)	6.5
	Residual	23	7(2)	1.0
Leukemia	Calendering, 5 +	8	57(21)	3.6
	Tire curing, 15 +	8	50(18)	3.1
	Tire building, 5 +	12	26(7)	1.6
	Elevators, 5 +	4	46(29)	2.9
	Tubes, 5 +	4	40(20)	2.5
	Rubber fabrics, 0 +	4	55(28)	3.5
	Residual	38	16(3)	1.0

[a] Employment in work areas is mutally exclusive and hierarchical from the top.

[b] Rate/100,000 persons/year. Standardized by the direct method to the age-specific person-year distribution of all 13,570 persons in the cohort. Values in parentheses are standard errors.

The excess of skin cancer among tire assembly workers is quite strong and reasonably stable. These men have considerable exposure of the skin to solvents and to uncured rubber. A causal interpretation is reasonable.

An excess of leukemia was found in a number of unrelated departments. Most, but not all, of these departments have considerable exposure to solvents. Leukemia and solvent exposure have been associated in another group of rubber workers.[22] Even though a causal interpretation seems reasonable, the specific solvent or solvents that is responsible is unknown. The prudent course is to reduce exposure to all solvents.

D. Comment

The three studies used as examples in this section utilized information from three different sources: medical absence records, disability retirement records, and hospital tumor registries. As in mortality studies, where death certificates are used in the measurement of disease, these records were collected for other reasons. However, each of these sources of information is of value to the occupational epidemiologist.

The development of morbidity systems within industry should capture these and other sources of morbidity data. Since this information has been collected for other purposes, it may not be ideally suited for epidemiologic purposes. One of the roles of the occupational epidemiologist is to work with the persons who have primary responsibility for these data so that their usefulness can be maximized.

A model example is the cancer registry maintained by the Du Pont Company.[23] Rather than having to survey hospital tumor registries, the registry identifies cancer cases through company-maintained insurance plans. Using these data, morbidity rates of cancer can be compared between the various groups of Du Pont employees. A logical extension of this system is to collect data on other causes of morbidity.

REFERENCES

1. McGill, D. B. and Motto, J. D., An industrial outbreak of toxic hepatitis due to methylenedianiline, *N. Engl. J. Med.*, 291, 278, 1974.
2. Kopelman, H., Robertson, M. H., and Sanders, P. G., The Epping jaundice, *Br. Med. J.*, 1, 514, 1966.
3. Olivier, N. E., Chloracne, *Arch. Dermatol.*, 99, 127, 1969.
4. Oliver, R. M., Toxic effects of 2,3,7,8 tetrachlorodibenzo 1,4 dioxin in laboratory workers, *Br. J. Ind. Med.*, 32, 49, 1975.
5. Whorton, D., Krauss, R. M., Marshall, S., and Milby, T. H., Infertility in male pesticide workers, *Lancet*, 2, 1259, 1977.
6. Wegman, D. H., Boden, L., and Levenstein, C., Health hazard surveillance by industrial workers, *Am. J. Public Health*, 65, 26, 1975.
7. Mantel, N. and Haenszel, W., Statistical aspects of the analysis of data from retrospective studies of disease, *J. Nat. Cancer Inst.*, 22, 719, 1959.
8. Hoover, R. and Cole, P., Temporal aspects of occupational bladder carcinogenesis, *N. Engl. J. Med.*, 288, 1040, 1973.
9. Cole, P., Hoover, R., and Friedell, G. H., Occupation and cancer of the lower urinary tract, *Cancer*, 29, 1250, 1972.
10. Cole, P., Monson, R. R., Haning, H., and Friedell, G. H., Smoking and cancer of the lower urinary tract, *N. Engl. J. Med.*, 284, 129, 1971.
11. Anthony, H. M. and Thomas, G. M., Tumors of the urinary bladder: an analysis of the occupations of 1030 patients in Leeds, England, *J. Nat. Cancer Inst.*, 45, 879, 1970.
12. Wynder, E. L. and Goldsmith, R., The epidemiology of bladder cancer — a second look, *Cancer*, 40, 1246, 1977.
13. Fine, L. J. and Peters, J. M., Respiratory morbidity in rubber workers. I. Prevalence of respiratory symptoms and disease in curing workers, *Arch. Environ. Health*, 31, 5, 1976.
14. Fine, L. J. and Peters, J. M., Respiratory morbidity in rubber workers. II. Pulmonary function in curing workers, *Arch. Environ. Health*, 31, 10, 1976.
15. Sidor, R. and Peters, J. M., Prevalence rates of chronic non-specific respiratory disease in fire fighters, *Am. Rev. Respir. Dis.*, 109, 255, 1974.
16. Peters, J. M., Theriault, G. P., Fine, L. F., and Wegman, D. M., Chronic effect of fire fighting on pulmonary function, *N. Engl. J. Med.*, 291, 1320, 1974.
17. Vital and Health Statistics Series, National Center for Health Statistics, Department of Health, Education and Welfare, Rockville, Md., periodic.
18. Monson, R. R., Duodenal ulcer as a second disease, *Gastroenterology*, 59, 712, 1970.
19. Tabershaw/Cooper Associates, A Morbidity Study of Petroleum Refinery Workers, Rep. American Petroleum Institute, Washington, D. C., April 28, 1975.
20. Lednar, W. M., Tyroler, H. A., McMichael, A. J., and Shy, C. M., The occupational determinants of chronic disabling pulmonary disease in rubber workers, *J. Occup. Med.*, 19, 263, 1977.
21. Monson, R. R. and Fine, L. J., Cancer mortality and morbidity among rubber workers, *J. Nat. Cancer Inst.*, 61, 1047, 1978.
22. McMichael, A. J., Spirtas, R., Kupper, L. L., and Gamble, J. F., Solvent exposure and leukemia among rubber workers: an epidemiologic study, *J. Occup. Med.*, 17, 234, 1975.
23. Pell, S., O'Berg, M. T., and Karrh, B. W., Cancer epidemiologic surveillance in the Du Pont Company, *J. Occup. Med.*, 20, 725, 1978.

Chapter 8
SURVEYS OF THE HEALTH STATUS OF EMPLOYED PERSONS

I. INTRODUCTION

In Chapters 6 and 7, mortality studies and morbidity studies have been discussed. These types of studies have until now been the usual types of epidemiologic studies carried out to assess the effects of the work place on employed persons.

However, ongoing epidemiologic evaluation of employee health status is becoming an important part of an occupational health program. Routine epidemiologic data are being collected both to permit continuous monitoring of employee health and to enable detailed evaluation of specific occupational health problems, should they develop. Eventually the need for expensive ad hoc mortality or morbidity studies should be reduced as the data bases grow within employed populations. Hopefully, such ongoing programs will permit the detection of occupational health problems at an earlier stage than is presently being done.

Also, a person's occupation as a potential cause of illness is increasingly becoming apparent to epidemiologists and physicians who practice in nonoccupational settings. The importance of a complete occupational history is becoming part of routine medical practice. In studies conducted within the hospital setting, information on a person's occupations is as essential as information on a person's habits.

In this chapter several designs for the collection and analysis of data within occupational settings and within hospital settings are considered. These designs are illustrated with examples of ongoing studies.

II. EXPOSURE-BASED SURVEILLANCE OF EMPLOYEE POPULATIONS

In setting up an epidemiologic surveillance system within industry, several possibilities exist as to the detail of data to be collected. The simplest design is to abstract and analyze data from a sickness and accident insurance system. The diagnoses recorded are related to the work areas of the currently employed population. Such a system is essentially passive in that it relies almost totally upon data collected for other purposes, i.e., health insurance data and personnel data.

In an active program, the occupational epidemiologist would collect data specifically designed for her needs. In addition to collecting personnel data on work area, areal industrial hygiene information would be collected on levels of exposure to substances that may affect an employee's health. Data on disease from insurance sources would be supplemented with information from preemployment history and physical exams, from nonroutine visits to a physician, and from periodic medical evaluations.

Finally, the most comprehensive surveillance system would include personal sampling for exposures in the work place as well as periodic multiphasic screening of physiologic factors that may become altered prior to the development of ill health.

There is no clear dividing line between these three study designs, and the features of all three designs may be combined into one comprehensive system. However, the cost of implementing a system relying exclusively on data collected for other purposes is clearly less than the cost of a system in which extensive primary information is collected on individual employees. The decision as to which type of system to implement depends upon the potential hazards in a given plant, upon the size of the plant, and upon the resources available.

A. Monitoring of Sickness and Accident Records

1. Collection of Data

In a system based on sickness and accident records, routine comparisons are made of disease rates among persons working in different areas. In order to make these comparisons, information on exposure and disease is needed for each individual in the work force.

It is logical to conduct such comparisons at some regular interval, say every year. From personnel records, information on an employee's work history can be obtained. Ideally, this information would include all employment data both during and prior to the year being evaluated. Practically speaking, however, it may be sufficient to determine only the person's department of employment on January 1 of the year being studied. Unless there is rapid movement from one department to another, each person's job at the beginning of the year should, in general, provide a reasonable measure of the pattern of employment for that year.

Information on disease will usually be more complex, since an individual may have more than one disease during the year. From insurance data, the diagnosis for each individual should be obtained. This assumes that such information is maintained in some usable form.

Information on potential confounding factors will usually be limited to basic demographic data, such as age, sex, and possibly ethnic derivation.

Selection or observation bias would not seem to be a problem in such surveys, if it can be assumed that health insurance claims are made or paid for valid medical reasons. It would seem unlikely that persons in one work area would selectively seek and gain compensation for a given condition.

2. Analysis of Data

The basic measure used to relate disease to exposure in this type of survey is the attack rate. For each department, the attack rate of each disease is computed by dividing the number of persons with a disease by the total number in the department. Because age is usually related to the rate of disease, it would be preferable to compute rates that are standardized for age by the direct method. The age distribution of the entire population is a reasonable standard to use. If desired, the rate can also be standardized for sex and ethnicity. Alternatively, age-standardized rates can be computed separately for each sex-ethnic group.

Since each individual may have more than one disease during a given year, she may appear more than once in the numerator of a disease rate. If the diseases are essentially independent, this would create no difficulty in interpretation of the data. However, there may be two diseases that are interrelated, such as bronchitis and pneumonia. To avoid the appearance that more than one illness is related to a specific work area, a reasonable approach would be to combine such similar diseases into a "respiratory disease" rubric.

On occasion, it may be apparent that it is misleading to define exposure simply as a person's job at the beginning of the year. There may be illnesses that develop acutely if a person transfers from one department to another. In this event it would be necessary to obtain information on each job a person held during a year as well as the dates of both transfers and diseases. A person could be counted more than once, both in the numerator and in the denominator of disease rates in specific departments. Considerable disentangling of specific diseases and specific exposures may be necessary. In such a situation, however, most causal associations should be apparent on clinical grounds.

On other occasions, it may be necessary to obtain a person's work history in the years preceding that being examined. There may be exposures that lead to diseases many years later, and simply using a current work history may lead to random misclassification of exposure. Since there must be some suspicion that such a situation exists, the most logical approach would be to do a case-control study of the disease that is suspected of being related to some work area. Controls might be a random or matched sample of persons with other diagnoses.

3. Interpretation of Data

As suggested above, one problem in interpreting associations based on a person's work experience at a point in time is random misclassification. Any real association between department and disease may be diluted because of the imprecise measure of exposure. However, no false association would be expected to arise because of this imprecision. Random misclassification is the price paid for the economy of the system.

If an association between a department and a disease is seen, assuming that age, sex, and ethnicity have been controlled, the meaning of the association is not usually obvious. If rates in only two departments are being compared, it is not known whether the high one is too high or the low one is too low. However, if out of ten departments one has a markedly elevated rate of a specific disease, a causal interpretation must be considered.

Tests of statistical significance have some role in such comparisons, in that the stability of any excess can be assessed. However, if the rates of many diseases are being computed among workers of many departments, some associations will be statistically significant simply because of random variation. Interpretation of associations must go beyond the presence or absence of statistical significance.

B. Active Epidemiologic Surveillance Systems

1. Collection of Data

The development of computer-based systems to collect and utilize data on employed persons is currently underway in American industry.[1-6] Increasingly it is becoming recognized that clinical reports and ad hoc morbidity and mortality studies are insufficient to protect the health of the worker. Also, governmental regulations are being developed that will require the maintenance of data on employed persons for at least 40 years after leaving employment.[7]

Collection of data for such a system logically begins at the time of initial employment and continues until death. Since the development and maintenance of such systems are expensive, careful consideration must be given not only to which data are collected but also to what use the data may be put. While vast amounts of data can potentially be included in such a system, it is far more important that useful data be collected.

Three basic types of data are needed here as in all epidemiologic studies: data on exposure, data on health status, and data on potentially confounding factors. One other feature is essential: maintenance and access to the source documents upon which the epidemiologic system is based. If attention is given to these four needs, an epidemiologic surveillance system in an industrial setting can be both useful and economic.

An epidemiologic surveillance system should *not* be designed so as to contain in active machine-readable storage all available data on exposure and health status. The cost of such a system would be prohibitive. Further, the utility of housing vast amounts of data is questionable, because much of the data will never be analyzed. Also, inasmuch as it is difficult to predict today what will be essential tomorrow, even comprehensive systems may fail to include critical elements.

An epidemiologic surveillance system *should* be designed to collect readily available information in summary form on exposure and disease. Important occupational health problems should be detectible under such a system. So long as the system permits ready access to details that may be needed in the future, no important information is lost. Ad hoc studies will still be necessary in certain situations.

a. Data on Exposure

Exposure data are of two general types: environmental and personal. Each type should be maintained essentially independently, but there should be a simple mechanism to link these data for analysis.

Environmental data should contain information on factors in the work place to which workers may be exposed. For a given work area, data should be maintained on which substances were used, how much was used, and the period of use. A reasonable method would be to record these data each year for each work area. The definition of work area will differ from plant to plant. It should be some identifiable area that is small enough to have relatively uniform usage of and exposure to industrial substances but large enough to have reasonable numbers of workers. Further, a work area should be convertible to some personnel code, so that data on work areas can be linked to data on individual workers.

In addition to the substances used in a work area, some information should be obtained periodically on the level of exposure to these substances. The amount of such industrial hygiene data will depend upon the level of exposure, the known toxicity and ease of measurement of the substances, and the number of persons exposed. Industrial hygiene data may result from areal sampling or from personal sampling. Each of these sources of data should be viewed as information on the work area rather than information on individual workers. Personal samples tend to reflect typical exposure patterns rather than data on individuals. For epidemiologic purposes, unless personal samples are taken for each worker in an area, these data are better treated as environmental data.

Finally, information should be maintained on the known or suspected effects on health of these substances. Such information should be updated as it becomes available. If different substances may have similar adverse health effects, some method is necessary to link persons exposed to these substances.

Personal data on exposure should contain information on where in a plant a person has worked, when she worked there, and what she did. *Where* a person worked should be coded using the same work area scheme as used in maintaining data on environmental exposures; ideally, the coding system provides a direct link to the system used for personnel purposes. *When* a person worked is necessary so as to measure length of exposure to an area as well as to determine whether a person was exposed at some specific time period. The details on *what* a person did may only be approximate. At a minimum, some information should be available as to whether a person was in a heavily or minimally exposed job within the work area.

Updating of personal data should be done periodically, perhaps every year. Either a person is in the same work area as the preceding year or has moved to another area. Although an annual updating will not record the details of a person who changes work area several times during a year, it is questionable whether it is necessary to accumulate such detailed information. Any association between work and disease that will be detected by an epidemiologic surveillance system will usually reflect the effects of relatively long-term exposures. The effects of short-term exposures are more likely to be acute and to be detected by clinical means. Certainly, if a worker population is exposed to many hazardous environments, more frequent updating of work history is indicated. But for routine purposes, an annual updating would seem to be sufficient.

b. Data on Health Status

At a preemployment medical examination, information is obtained on demographic characteristics, work history habits, family history of disease and past or present illnesses in the individual. Diseases ascertained at this point should be considered to be potential confounding factors, because they have occurred prior to employment.

Illnesses or abnormalities in health status that occur subsequent to employment might have occurred because of work exposures or for other reasons. The purpose of an epidemiologic surveillance system is to assist in determining the reason for these illnesses.

Abnormalities in health status may be detected either before clinical illness develops, at the stage of frank disease, or at death. Preclinical disease is detected either through medical screening programs or through routine medical examinations. Not all of preclinical disease is likely to progress to clinical disease. Clinical disease, including accidents, may be diagnosed by a visit to a health facility maintained by an employer or to some other medical facility. Whether the information on outside medical visits is accessible to an occupational surveillance system depends to some extent upon local medical practice as well as on medical insurance schemes. Information on death may not be available for persons who die many years after termination of employment. Thus the nature and extent of data available on employee health status will vary from person to person, from plant to plant, and from industry to industry.

At a minimum, an epidemiologic surveillance system should contain information on cause of death. Death certificates are public records and are usually routinely obtained by a company for insurance purposes. Death benefit plans usually cover active workers and those who are employed long enough to earn vested rights. Persons who work only a few years and who terminate employment usually are not followed. However, it is possible to determine whether a death claim has been filed for these persons through the Social Security Administration (see Chapter 6). Also, plans for a National Death Index are currently underway; it will be possible to determine whether an individual is known to have died in the U.S. by submitting her name to the Index.

Information on diseases that develop between retirement and death will usually not be available. While such illnesses could be the result of occupational exposures, the cost of obtaining this information would seem to be prohibitive. Any important disease which occurs during this period will usually be mentioned on the death certificate.

Inasmuch as most industries maintain sickness and accident insurance for their employees, information on most important illnesses can be obtained from these sources. It is important that there be communication between the insurance personnel and the epidemiologist within a company so that the data that an epidemiologist needs is collected and coded by the insurance program. At a minimum, the disease for which an insurance claim is made should be coded using some standard system, such as the International Classification of Diseases.[8] An annual updating of diseases from the insurance file would seem to be reasonable.

Whereas diseases for which insurance claims are paid tend to be of some minimum severity and subject to some external scrutiny, diseases diagnosed only in routine medical practice are much more variable. There is a wide variation in the propensity of individuals to visit physicians; there is variation in the diagnostic procedures used by physicians, and there is variation in the diagnoses given to symptom complexes. Information on disease, whether it is collected by physicians employed by industry or employed elsewhere, may be subject to both selection and observation biases. Groups of individuals within a given work area may be more prone to seek medical attention for some minor illness than groups from other work areas. The rate of diagnosed illness will obviously be affected by this bias. If a disease is suspected of being the result of some exposure, persons with that exposure may be more carefully monitored for disease. Also, the criteria used to categorize a worker as diseased or nondiseased may differ among work areas with different exposures.

The above problems exist to a greater extent for information obtained in periodic medical examinations. Since routine checkups are largely voluntary, it is quite likely that persons who have annual exams have exposure or disease patterns that differ from persons who do not see a physician each year.

Great care must therefore be exercised in entering data from routine medical practice into an epidemiologic surveillance system. If information on visits for illnesses is to be entered, there should be some assurance that all members of the employee population have equal access to and use of medical care. If information on routine health maintenance examinations is to be entered, such examinations should be carried out on everyone in some defined employee population.

c. Data on Confounding Factors

In collecting data on exposure and disease in an employed population, primary emphasis must be placed on the prevention of selection and observation bias. Once data biased for these reasons are entered, no amount of analysis can correct the false associations that may arise.

However, in all nonexperimental epidemiologic data, associations between exposure and disease are likely to occur because of confounding bias. While some of these associations can be prevented by matching, such a strategy is not realistic in a surveillance system. Therefore, an effort must be made to collect as much relevant information on confounding factors as possible. In determining whether a specific factor is relevant, it should be kept in mind that in order for a factor to be confounding, it must be associated both with exposure and disease.

Much information on potential confounding factors can be obtained at the preemployment examination. Examples of data to be collected include previous and current medical conditions, habits such as smoking, drinking and diet, demographic characteristics such as age, sex, ethnicity, educational level, place of residence, and previous work history.

Subsequent information on confounding factors need be collected only infrequently and only for factors that are likely to change, such as habits. Every 5 years would seem to be a realistic interval for obtaining information on confounding factors.

The purpose of obtaining information on confounding factors is to be able to control for confounding if an association is seen between some exposure or work area and some disease. Therefore, some thought should be given to how likely it is that a given factor may be confounding. While most of the factors listed above are likely to relate to the rate of disease, it is less certain that they will be associated with exposure. Further, even if a factor is confounding, it may account for only a fraction of any association between exposure and disease. Therefore, in recording information on confounding factors, some balance should be kept between what is possible and what is likely.

d. Recording of Data vs. Coding of Data

Vast amounts of data can be accumulated in an employed population on exposures, diseases, and confounding factors. A major challenge to the occupational epidemiologist is to develop a realistic surveillance system that is comprehensive yet economical.

A key feature of such a system is that not all data that are recorded need be coded. A large portion of the data collected will be useful only in specific situations, and the routine coding and computer processing of such data are not necessary. However, if this strategy is to be followed, it is essential that the recorded data be maintained in a readily accessible format.

The source documents for an epidemiologic surveillance system are personnel records, purchase and use records, medical records, and insurance records. In these documents are contained a person's complete work history, the substances used in the plant, the medical information on employees, and the benefits and payments made through insurance. These are the daily working records of an organization and are not developed or designed for epidemiologic purposes. Nevertheless, it is important that these records not be destroyed when they become outdated but that they be stored for future epidemiologic use.

An epidemiologic surveillance system obtains most of its information from these source documents. The source documents provide the complete records on exposure and disease, but they are not suitable for active monitoring of health. An epidemiologic surveillance system, on the other hand, need not be complete but should be designed to be useful on a day-to-day basis.

Because needs will differ from industry to industry, from plant to plant, and from time to time, no absolute rules can be set down as to what information should be entered into a surveillance system. However, data on the following factors would seem to be necessary:

1. Environmental exposure
      Substances used in each work area
      Concentrations in air of known or suspected hazardous substances
2. Personal exposure
      Work area experience
      Nature of job within work area
3. Health status
      Major diseases requiring hospitalization
      Chronic diseases
      Cause of death
4. Confounding factors
      Routine demographic data (age, ethnicity, sex)
      Habits (smoking, drinking)
      Previous major illnesses
      Previous work history

Data on confounding factors should be updated perhaps every five years; data on the other factors should be updated perhaps annually.

Routine coding for active computer usage probably is not necessary for all of the industrial hygiene measurements that are routinely made. Routine coding is not needed for all of the detailed medical information obtained during routine medical examinations. An epidemiologic surveillance system should be designed to detect relatively major problems in fairly large groups of employees; such a system is unlikely to be sensitive enough under any circumstances to detect minor medical problems among small numbers of persons.

In this section I have concentrated upon what I believe to be important features of data collection for epidemiologic surveillance systems in industry. I have not considered whether other uses may be made of the data available in source documents. For example, detailed computer processing of industrial hygiene data may be desired for technical reasons, or detailed coding of medical records may be desired for medical care purposes. Clearly, the setting up of a computer based information system on health involves more than epidemiologic concerns. However, it is important that the needs of the epidemiologist and the limitations of epidemiologic data are kept in mind, so that an expensive, cumbersome system not be needlessly developed.

These comments are based primarily on general considerations of epidemiology rather than on specific knowledge of occupational medicine practice. Only through experience and through the cooperation of industrial hygienists, physicians, and epidemiologists can reasonable functioning surveillance systems be developed.

2. Analysis of Data

The basic measure used to relate disease to exposure in this type of survey is the incidence (or mortality) rate. For each work area, the incidence rate of disease is computed by dividing the number of persons with a disease by the person-years of follow-up after initial exposure to a work area. As in the analysis of data from sickness and accident records, age-standardized rates should be computed, possibly within each sex and ethnicity group.

The analysis of data from an ongoing epidemiologic surveillance system in general is more complicated than the analysis of data from sickness and accident records. A person is followed over time, may have many different exposure experiences, and may have many different diseases that occur at different times. These data are similar to those obtained in mortality studies, yet are even more complex. Illness may occur at any stages of life whereas death occurs only once. External death rates are available for comparison purposes in mortality studies, but the analysis of morbidity rates must be based almost entirely on within-plant experience.

In setting up a program to analyze data from an ongoing surveillance system, the simplest analyses should be done first. These would be the same as the analyses done using sickness and accident data — annual attack rates of disease would be computed for persons employed in a work area at the beginning of each year. If work-related illnesses are detected at this phase of analysis, the illnesses would likely be acute diseases following relatively short exposures.

Another screening analysis would be to compare age-standardized incidence rates of disease over a period of years among all persons who ever worked in a given area, irrespective of whether they currently are working there. Any disease occurring between entrance into a work area and the present would be counted in the numerator; the denominator would be the person-years between entrance and the present. Analyses of this nature would not be independent, because persons may have more than one work area exposure and more than one disease. The disentangling of these nonindependent data is largely an ad hoc procedure — an excess of a disease in a specific work area could be causal or could be due to confounding by a second work area.

Also, at this stage, a population can be stratified into levels of exposure to a work area on the basis of years worked in the area. The data can be analysed to determine whether persons who worked for a relatively long time in the area had more disease than those who worked a short time. In such an analysis, care must be taken in the apportioning of person-years (See Chapter 6). Work-related illnesses of a chronic nature should be detectable by this type of analysis.

Analyses such as these can also be directed to investigate the possible association of a specific disease and a specific exposure. The work force can be divided into two groups — those with the exposure or work experience of interest and all other persons. Computation of two age-standardized incidence rates of the disease of interest may be the only analysis needed. As above, stratification of the exposed persons into levels of years worked may be carried out.

At some point, the amount of information contained in an epidemiologic surveillance system may be insufficient to investigate fully some hypothesized or actual association. It may be necessary to do some ad hoc data collection by searching through the more detailed records of the past. It is at this point that an orderly system of maintaining old records is important. Either a case-control or a cohort strategy can be carried out. If the disease of interest is well-defined and the exposure information is incomplete, the personnel and environmental records can be searched for detailed information on exposure. Records would be searched for persons with the disease (cases) and for some sample of other persons (controls). Conversely, if additional medical information is needed, the medical records of exposed and a sample of nonexposed persons can be searched.

It might be argued that if complete data are not kept in computer-retrievable format, imprecise information will be all that is available for exposure and for disease, and that important associations will be missed because of random misclassification. While one can not predict how likely such situations may be, it seems unlikely that they would occur frequently. Epidemiology is an imprecise science, and there will be times when true associations are not detected as quickly as might be possible.

3. Interpretation of Data

A central problem in the interpretation of associations in epidemiologic screening programs in industry will probably be due to the large amount of data that will be available. The numbers of exposures and combinations of exposures will be large as will be the numbers of medical conditions. Because of the normal variability of epidemiologic data, there will be strong, positive, statistically significant associations seen that simply are not interpretable. Also, the absolute size of any disease rate will have no inherent meaning or outside standard of comparison.

In such a situation it is essential that there be ready communication among industrial groups as to the results of their analyses. Comparison from time to time and from place to place must become routine, so that an opinion can be formed as to the generalizibility of any single association. This will require both some relaxation of industry concern for privacy and for governmental concern for regulation. Industry should not fear to let others know about tentative associations between exposures and disease, and government should not base regulations on tenuous associations. Rather than the two parties behaving as adversaries, some methods should be developed for the rapid and reasoned transmission and interpretation of epidemiologic data from occupational groups.

C. Multiphasic Screening Programs

In a detailed occupational epidemiology program designed to measure associations between exposure and disease, extensive information on individuals would be collected on exposures and on measures of health status. There would be routine periodic sampling from the work environment and routine periodic screening for disease and precursors of disease.

Sampling from the environment would usually be directed at some specific toxic substance. Presumably some maximum level of exposure would be permissible, and the industrial hygiene sampling would be aimed at keeping personal exposure at safe levels. These data could also be used for epidemiologic purpose.

Measurement of health status would indicate routine examinations such as chest X-rays, pulmonary function tests, urinalyses, a battery of blood measurements and possible other screening procedures such as cytology or radiography. These screening tests would be aimed at detecting preclinical disease, such as early cancer, so that treatment can be initiated early in the disease process.

Clearly, such intensive screening programs are expensive and cannot be carried out as a matter of routine. Further, the utility of many screening programs has been questioned.[9] Whether the early detection of, say, lung cancer leads to any overall improvement in a person's health status has yet to be demonstrated unequivocally.

Screening for epidemiologic purposes must be kept separate from screening for medical purposes. On a population basis, mass screening is expensive and of questionable utility. In other words, the cost may be far greater than any potential benefit. However, it may be the judgment of an occupational physician that screening of a selected group of employees is indicated. It may be her judgment that the potential benefit is great enough to offset any cost, no matter how great. For example, it seems logical to provide periodic screening examinations of urine cytology for persons who have worked for long periods of time with bladder carcinogens. Such examinations are part of humane medical practice and need not be influenced by scientific epidemiologic considerations. The practice of medicine and the practice of epidemiology are both imperfect, and the judgments of the individual physician or epidemiologist must count as much as the dogma of the profession.

Data on health from a multiphasic screening program may be treated essentially as data from an active epidemiologic surveillance system. Abnormal outcomes can be treated as diseases and related to work exposures. Also, these data should be used in the evaluation of multiphasic screening programs. As time goes by and as frank clinical disease develops, it will be important to relate data from screening tests to data from subsequent disease. Such analyses should be done to assess whether there is any relationship between an abnormal screening test and the later development of disease. It is important to evaluate not only the relationship between occupational exposures and disease, but also the system used to collect data on that relationship.

D. Example — Rubber Workers
1. Collection of Data

In 1975 patterns of morbidity were assessed among active employees at seven B. F. Goodrich rubber plants.[10] Two sources of data on health were used: sickness and accident insurance claims between 1/1/73 and 10/31/74 and a questionnaire mailed to 10,933 active employees. In addition, a person's department of employment as of 9/1/74 was determined.

No precise information on disease diagnosis was available from the insurance claims. Rather, a rough designation of reason for the claim was specified, e.g., circulatory disease, respiratory disease, etc. On the mailed questionnaire, a variety of questions were asked about current or past signs and symptoms of ill health and about specific illnesses. Also, information was obtained on past employment and on current smoking patterns.

Obtaining response to the mail questionnaire was difficult. Even though there was active support for this effort by national and local union leaders, there was only a 57% response after three mailings.

2. Analysis of Data and Results

Initially, the data were analyzed in three ways: questionnaire data only, insurance data only, and a combination of the two. Because of the imprecision of the diagnosis in the insurance data, subsequent analyses were done either on the questionnaire data or on a combination of the two sources. In analyzing the combined data, a person was considered to have a disease if he or she had a specific category of disease listed in the insurance data and if he or she responded "yes" to a specific question relating to that disease.

Table 8.1

CRUDE AND AGE-ADJUSTED[a] PERCENTAGES OF PERSONS WITH CANCER
ACCORDING TO PLANT: NONBLACK MALES ONLY

Plant	Total number	Disease according to questionnaire			Disease according to both questionnaire and insurance		
		Number	Crude %	Adjusted %[a]	Number	Crude %	Adjusted %[a]
A.	1177	42	3.6	2.5	16	1.4	0.8
B.	841	7	0.8	2.5	3	0.4	1.6
C.	271	8	3.7	3.1	3	1.4	1.0
D.	171	1	0.6	0.8	0	0	0
E.	1113	42	3.8	3.9	8	0.7	0.7
F.	854	27	3.2	2.6	4	0.5	0.3
G.	842	49	5.8	5.7	4	0.5	0.5
All	5215	176	3.4	—	38	0.7	—

[a] Adjusted by the direct method to the age distribution of all 5215 employees who responded to the questionnaire.

Table 8.2

CRUDE AND AGE-ADJUSTED[a] PERCENTAGES OF PERSONS WITH
CIRCULATORY DISEASE ACCORDING TO PLANT; NONBLACK MALES
ONLY

Plant	Total	Disease according to questionnaire			Disease according to both questionnaire and insurance		
		Number	Crude %	Adjusted %	Number	Crude %	Adjusted %[a]
A.	1177	516	43.8	38.6	57	4.8	3.5
B.	841	287	34.1	44.9	11	1.3	4.9
C.	271	100	46.1	42.7	14	6.5	5.1
D.	171	71	41.5	44.1	5	2.9	3.9
E.	1113	499	44.8	44.8	63	5.7	5.6
F.	854	381	44.6	42.0	71	8.3	7.0
G.	842	358	42.5	42.4	43	5.1	5.8
All	5215	2,212	42.4	—	264	5.1	—

[a] Adjusted by the direct method to the age distribution of all 5215 employees who responded to the questionnaire.

Crude and age-adjusted rates of disease were computed according to plant and according to department of employment. These rates could best be thought of as prevalence rates of persons with a history of having or having had a disease. Age-adjustment was necessary because disease rates were higher in older persons and because the age distribution differed among workers in different plants and in different departments.

Examples of the data collected are presented in Tables 8.1 to 8.4. As might be expected among a group of actively employed persons, the rate of cancer was low. There was poor correlation between a report of cancer on the questionnaire and on the insurance claim. Of the 176 occurrences of cancer reported on the questionnaire, only 38 were also reported on the insurance claim.

As can be seen from Table 8.1, there were too few persons with cancer to permit an assessment of the association of cancer with plant. If only data from the questionnaire are evaluated, the rate in plant G is quite a bit higher than the rate in other plants.

Table 8.3

CRUDE AND AGE-ADJUSTED[a] PERCENTAGES OF PERSONS WITH CIRCULATORY
DISEASE ACCORDING TO WORK AREA; NONBLACK MALES ONLY

Work area	Total number	Disease according to questionnaire			Disease according to both questionnaire and insurance		
		Number	Crude %	Adjusted %	Number	Crude %	Adjusted %
Engineering	745	328	44.0	39.8	54	7.2	5.7
Aerospace	76	31	40.8	35.5	3	3.9	2.2
Warehouse/shipping	231	100	43.3	41.7	14	6.1	5.5
Shops	144	52	36.1	26.0	6	4.2	2.4
Processing	690	309	44.8	45.5	36	5.2	5.7
Chemical	106	62	58.5	44.8	6	5.7	8.0
Tires, misc.	604	276	45.6	43.9	39	6.5	5.6
Tire building	1654	616	37.2	41.1	69	4.2	5.6
Tire curing	486	223	45.9	45.0	22	4.5	4.4
Misc. industrial products	194	82	42.3	46.1	3	1.5	2.6
Hose/belt	203	90	44.3	48.2	8	3.9	6.7
All	5215	2212	42.4	—	264	5.1	—

[a] Adjusted by the direct method to the age distribution of the 5215 employees who responded to the questionnaire.

Table 8.4

CRUDE AND AGE-ADJUSTED[a] PERCENTAGES OF
SPECIFIC SYMPTOMS ON THE QUESTIONNAIRE IN
WORKERS IN SPECIFIC DEPARTMENTS; NONBLACK
AKRON MALES ONLY

Type of symptom	Department	Total number	Disease according to questionnaire:		
			Number	Crude %	Adjusted %[a]
Headache	Warehouse	27	6	22.2	15.7
	Other	1150	205	17.8	17.4
Cardiac	Warehouse	27	1	3.7	4.8
	Other	1150	225	19.7	19.2
Skin	Processing	50	29	58.0	48.5
	Other	1127	465	41.3	40.8
Back	Tire building	149	50	33.6	33.4
	Other	1028	319	31.0	30.6
Hearing loss	Tire curing	26	8	30.8	17.1
	Other	1151	261	22.7	22.5
Respiratory	Processing	26	7	26.9	16.3
	Tire curing	50	9	18.0	20.0
	Other	1101	196	17.8	17.3

[a] Adjusted by the direct method to the age distribution of all 1177 Akron employees who responded to the questionnaire.

However, when the joint data from the questionnaire and the insurance claims are considered, no such excess is seen.

As can be seen in Tables 8.2 and 8.3, over 42% of persons reported one or more symptoms relating to the circulatory system. However, insurance claims were paid for only 12% (264/2212) of these persons during the period of the study. While considerably more persons reported circulatory disease than cancer, the data are equally difficult to evaluate. The rates by plant differ only slightly. Among work area, the chemical department has a higher rate when the joint questionnaire-insurance data are considered, but has essentially an average rate according to the questionnaire.

In Table 8.4 are presented rates for six specific symptoms reported on the questionnaire. These symptoms were selected because of an *a priori* judgment that they might be more prevalent among workers in the specific departments. As can be seen, there was little evidence to suggest that the *a priori* notions were correct.

3. Interpretation of Data

The description of this study is not presented as a model for an occupational epidemiologist. Collecting data through a mail questionnaire is less preferable than collecting data through some ongoing surveillance program. While collecting data through health and sickness insurance claims will likely prove to be useful, this system was in its infancy. A major shortcoming was in the way diagnoses were recorded. Since the system was set up with no intention of being used for epidemiologic purposes, an imprecise scheme was adopted for coding diagnoses.

However, the data are not atypical of data that will be collected in epidemiologic surveillance systems within industry. Cancer will appear with low frequency inasmuch as it is primarily a disease of older persons. It remains to be seen whether preclinical cancer can be detected and treated successfully. Diseases such as cardiovascular disease will probably occur with a relatively high frequency, since many of its symptoms occur in many people. However, most cardiovascular disease is probably due to nonoccupational reasons, and it is questionable whether any small risk imparted by occupation can be detected against the background of a much larger risk imparted by lifestyle.

Even though excess rates of disease are seen, it is never straightforward to determine the reason for the excess. It must be kept in mind that the data derive from a nonexperimental process and that health status is undoubtedly related to reason for employment. If persons with mild cardiovascular disease are assigned to a given work area, the rate of subsequent cardiovascular disease will probably be higher in that area.

As epidemiologic surveillance systems are developed and time passes, large amounts of data will accumulate. While analyses of these data will be relatively straightforward, interpretation will be difficult.

III. DISEASE-BASED SURVEILLANCE OF HOSPITALIZED PERSONS

Exposure-based surveillance within industrial populations may be thought of as cohort studies. The initial information obtained is on one's occupation or exposure. As time passes, information on disease accumulates. Such systems are useful in that they can collect data on a variety of illnesses in a well-defined population that is relatively disease-free at its definition. However, these systems tend to be narrow in the spectrum of occupational exposure.

A disease-based exposure system has fewer limits on the potential occupational exposure in the persons surveyed. Hospitalized persons come from a wide variety of occupational backgrounds and may represent a wide variety of hazardous exposures. This breadth, however, limits the utility of disease-based systems. It is likely that many factors contribute to the etiology of most diseases, and that for any disease occupational factors contribute to only a small percentage of the cases. Unless an occupation is relatively common in a given geographic area, the percentage of occupationally-induced disease will be very low in a group of hospital patients. It is necessary, therefore, to focus disease-based surveillance on areas where specific industries are relatively common.

Two basic types of methods may be used in collecting data on hospitalized persons. The greatest detail on occupational history and on personal habits can be obtained in an interview study. However, the cost per patient is very high and not suited to exploratory surveillance systems. On the other hand, the cost of reviewing hospital records is relatively low, so that many records can be reviewed for relatively low cost. However, the information on occupation and on potential confounding factors is usually quite limited in hospital records. Record systems are best suited to exploratory studies where data on large numbers of persons are needed; interview studies are preferable when detailed information is desired on relatively specific hypotheses.

A. Record Review Studies

The cause of many congenital malformations is unknown; the cause of many abnormalities of pregnancy is unknown; the effects of parental occupation on the mother and fetus during pregnancy are unknown. To evaluate the association between these factors, we are conducting a case-control study in the Akron, Ohio area.[11] A high proportion of men and women who live in this area have been employed in the rubber industry.

In choosing the type of epidemiologic study to use in evaluating this association, both cohort and case-control designs were considered. While the occurrence of abnormalities of pregnancies, including birth defects, overall is relatively high, perhaps 10 to 20%, the rates of specific abnormalities are low — perhaps 1/1000. Therefore, it would have been necessary to follow a large number of male and female rubber workers and comparison workers in order to assemble sufficient cases of disease for analysis. A cohort study done prospectively would have to proceed for many years. A cohort assembled from past company records would have to be very large.

In considering whether a case-control study may be preferable, an important consideration was the prevalence of persons with "exposure" — having worked in the rubber industry. If only a small percentage of persons in the Akron area had been rubber workers, it would have been necessary to identify a large number of cases (and controls) so that there would be a sufficient number of rubber workers. However, since the main industry in Akron is (or was) rubber manufacture, the percentage of rubber workers is high. In addition, by utilizing the diagnostic indices that are maintained by all hospitals, cases with abnormalities of pregnancy could be readily identified. Further, by selecting a sample of normal pregnancies, controls could be selected from the same information source as the cases.

1. Collection of Data

Cases and controls are being selected by a search of hospital diagnostic indices. Each time a person is discharged from a hospital, a code is assigned for each diagnoses. For mothers, codes are assigned for all medical conditions and conditions of pregnancy, including normal delivery. For children, codes are assigned for all abnormalities noted at or subsequent to delivery. Cases are all women and children with an abnormal diagnosis. Controls are a 20% sample of all women with the diagnosis of "normal delivery". They are being selected as all women whose hospital unit record number ends with a "1" or a "2". While this is a systematic rather than a random sample, the assignment of a unit record number is unlikely to be associated either with parental occupation or with outcome of pregnancy.

Diagnostic indices are being reviewed at four Akron area hospitals with obstetric services. Each of these hospitals has used the International Classification of Diseases (ICD) for some time. It is straightforward to abstract the desired diagnoses, since abnormalities of pregnancy are grouped together as are congenital malformations. The diagnostic indices are sorted in order of diagnosis, thus all diagnoses of interest are within a defined area of the index.

Prior to using the ICD, these hospitals used Standard Nomenclature.[12] Diagnoses coded under Standard are sorted according to organ system rather than diagnosis. Also, the logic behind this coding system is more complicated than that behind the ICD system. It is considerably more difficult and time-consuming to abstract desired diagnoses from the Standard files.

Selection of cases and controls is essentially free from selection bias or observation bias since no information on parental employment is available. Of course, it is possible that when the diagnoses were assigned by the physician for the mother or the child, there was a difference in the way codes were assigned for rubber working families than for nonrubber working families. While this possibility cannot be ruled out, it seems remote.

After all of the diagnostic codes have been abstracted along with the unit record numbers and the dates of hospitalization, the data are sorted by date, record number, and diagnosis. This results in a computer file that lists the diagnoses assigned in each year for each pregnancy.

Using these lists, data clerks locate the medical records and abstract the relevant data. This study is aimed at exploring whether associations exist between occupation and pregnancy rather than at elaborating upon a known association. Therefore, given a fixed amount of resources, the study is aimed at collecting a small amount of information on a large amount of persons rather than at collecting detailed information on a small population. In reviewing the medical record, only essential information that is readily available is abstracted. This information includes occupation of mother and of father, basic demographic data (ethnicity, religion, and years of schooling), basic data on the pregnancy (date of last menstrual period, age of mother, number and outcome of previous pregnancies), and basic information on the child (vital status, sex, birth-weight). Information on prenatal X-ray exposure and cigarette smoking habits of the mother are also sought, but frequently such information is not included. Little information on drugs used during pregnancy is available in the obstetric delivery record, and therefore it was judged not worth the time to search for such data.

2. Analysis of Data

The basic measure to be examined in these data is the percentage of mothers and of fathers who are or were rubber workers. At one extreme, the percentage in the cases may be compared to the percentage in the controls. However, since the cases comprise a variety of diagnoses, the percentage of parents who are rubber workers should be examined within each diagnostic category. The controls are all women with a normal delivery (or more generally, all normal pregnancies where both the pregnancy and the child are normal). A variety of case groups can be defined either mutually exclusively or overlapping. For example, one case group could be women with bleeding in pregnancy and a second could be women with first trimester bleeding only. A case group could be all malformed children (with malformations diagnosed at or shortly after birth), children with central nervous system malformations, or simply children with hydrocephaly. A large number of different case groups can be defined.

Each case group is compared to the controls with respect to parental employment in the rubber industry. If the percentage exposed is the same, the "exposure ratio", the odds ratio, and the rate ratio are all 1.0. If the percentages differ, the odds ratio may be computed as described in Chapter 4. This crude odds ratio is the basic measure of association between parental employment in the rubber industry and that particular abnormality.

Inasmuch as no data are yet available from this study, the utility of this approach is unknown. Clearly, information on occupation must be available in the medical record. Also, it is essential that the occupation of interest be relatively common in the geographic area being studied — say 10% or so. If this is not the case, it will be necessary to collect large amounts of data simply to have stable exposure rates among the case and controls. However, the cost of record review is much less than the cost of personal interviews.

B. Interview Studies

1. Conduct

The model for case-control surveillance comes from an ongoing program in drug epidemiology.[13,14] Patients in a number of hospitals are interviewed as to past and present usage of medications and as to a variety of potential confounding factors. Basic demographic characteristics of the patient are obtained from the medical record or from the patient.

In obtaining a drug history, patients are asked detailed questions about past usage. They are not simply asked whether they have ever used any drugs, nor are they asked whether they took one or more of a long list of specific drug products. Rather, they are asked questions of the form. "Did you ever take a medication for X?", where X is one of the medical conditions. If a person responds yes to any of the questions, details are obtained as to type or name of medication and dates, dosage and duration of use.

The interviews are conducted by nurse-monitors who are stationed permanently in one or more hospital wards. The nurse-monitors are part of the medical team, and there is no disruption of the hospital routine. Flexibility is built into the system in that priorities are assigned as to which diagnoses are most important. Patients with diagnoses in which there is special interest are interviewed in preference to patients with a lower priority diagnosis.

In any specific analysis, cases are persons with the disease of interest and controls are all other persons. It is important that controls comprise a variety of diagnoses, so that one can examine the percentage of exposure among the component diagnoses of the control group. If there is a causal association between exposure and disease, one would expect that the rate of exposure among the various components of the control group would vary little and would be less than the rate among the case group. If the controls are comprised of persons with only one diagnosis, it is difficult to determine whether the exposure among the cases is in excess or the exposure among the controls is in deficit.

Because of the nature of hospitalized persons, data analysis is usually not done on all cases and controls interviewed. Usually, the purpose of a study is to evaluate the association between a drug and a disease in otherwise healthy persons. Therefore, persons are excluded from both the case and the control series if they have medical conditions that are risk factors for the disease of interest. Also, persons who have previously been hospitalized for that illness usually are excluded. These groups of persons almost certainly have their illness for reasons not related to the drug or drugs being evaluated, and their presence makes it more difficult to detect an association, should one exist.

Also, if the drug being evaluated produces more than one disease, persons with these other diseases should be excluded from the controls. Such patients are in the hospital because of their drug-induced disease, and their presence artifically raises the percentage of exposure among the controls.

In analyzing data from case-control studies, either matched or unmatched analyses can be carried out. In a matched analyses one would select one or more controls per case. The controls would be matched to the cases or factors known to be confounding, e.g., age and sex. In an unmatched analysis, control for confounding would be carried out by a stratification procedure. Comparable results are usually obtained from the two general methods. The basic measure of association is the crude or Mantel-Haenszel standardized relative odds.

2. Example

In the case-control surveillance system described, the initial report presented the association between cigarette smoking and myocardial infarction in young women.[14] The data was derived from a study designed to evaluate the association between oral contraceptive use and myocardial infarction in women less than 50 years old. Because a heart attack is uncommon in young women, a network of 152 hospitals was set up. Whenever a woman aged 49 or less was admitted to one of these hospitals with definite or suspected myocardial infarction, an interview was conducted with women who survived the incident. For each potential case, 5 to 20 control interviews were conducted.

Between July 1976 and December 1977, 170 definite cases and 2775 controls were interviewed. An analysis was conducted of the relationship between cigarette smoking and myocardial infarction. There were 1451 controls who had diagnoses considered *a priori* to be related to cigarette smoking. These women were excluded from further consideration. Also excluded were cases and controls with prior medical conditions which were risk factors for myocardial infarction. There remained 55 cases and 843

Table 8.5
CIGARETTE SMOKING AMONG 843
CONTROLS ACCORDING TO DIAGNOSIS

Diagnosis	Number of patients	Cigarette smokers	
		Number	Percent
Musculoskeletal	191	97	51
Trauma	137	77	56
Abdominal conditions	163	93	57
Other	352	189	54

Table 8.6
PERCENTAGE DISTRIBUTION
OF POTENTIAL
CONFOUNDING FACTORS
AMONG 55 CASES AND 220
CONTROLS

Characteristic	Cases	Controls
White ethnicity	87	86
Nulliparous	24	25
Premenopausal	71	67
Education > 12 years	27	33

Table 8.7
PERCENTAGE DISTRIBUTION OF
CIGARETTE SMOKING AND
MYOCARDIAL INFARCTION IN 55
CASES AND 220 CONTROLS

Cigarettes/ day	Cases	Controls	Odds ratio
Never smoked	7	33	1.0
Ex-smokers	4	12	1.4
1—14	15	15	4.4
15—24	27	27	4.6
25—34	22	7	14
≥35	25	5	21

controls. As seen in Table 8.5, there was little variation among the controls in percentage of smokers.

To control potential confounding by age and hospital, four age-hospital matched controls were selected for each case. Confounding by a number of other factors was unlikely in that, as illustrated in Table 8.6, the factors were distributed similarly in the cases and in the controls.

As seen in Table 8.7, there was a clear-cut dose-response relationship between cigarette smoking and myocardial infarction. Women who were smoking 35 or more cigarettes/day had a risk of myocardial infarction that was 21 times that of women who had never smoked.

3. Extension to the Evaluation of Occupational Exposures

While these data were collected to evaluate the association between drugs and disease, they can be used to evaluate other associations. Instead of or in addition to collecting detailed drug histories, complete occupational histories could be obtained.

However, there are important differences between drugs and occupations to be considered in designing such studies. Drug usage is quite common, and over the course of a lifetime each person may be exposed to many drugs. All drugs are biologically active, and unwanted side effects are not uncommon. Further, there is not a great deal of variation in drug usage from place to place, and thus case-control surveillance for effects of drugs might be done in a variety of locations.

Occupations are much more geographically concentrated. While a given individual may have a number of occupations in her lifetime, many persons have only one or two. Further, many occupations are unlikely to have important effects on health. Therefore, if a case-control surveillance system were to be set up to monitor unwanted effects of occupations, careful selection of location is essential. Also, questions on potential occupational exposures must take into account the details of the common occupations present among the population served by the participating hospitals.

Case-control surveillance for unsuspected health effects of occupations is clearly less efficient than an epidemiologic surveillance system within an industry. However, in areas where small industries predominate and where no in-house epidemiologic surveillance system is present, it should offer a reasonable alternative in the collection of data relating occupation and disease. While it is unlikely to be an inexpensive way to search for totally unsuspected occupational disease, case-control surveillance should be of value in evaluating suspected associations. In such situations both the geographic location and the occupational history questions can be tailored to some specific inquiry.

REFERENCES

1. Hipp, L. L., Jirak, P. D., and Golonka, E. J., Evolution of an occupational health examination program, *J. Occup. Med.*, 19, 205, 1977.
2. Barrett, C. D. and Belk, H. D., A computerized occupational medical surveillance program, *J. Occup. Med.*, 19, 732, 1977.
3. Forbes, J. D., Dunn, J. P., Hillman, G., Hipp, L. L., McDonagh, T. J., Pell, S., and Reichwein, G. F., Utilization of medical information systems in American occupational medicine, *J. Occup. Med.*, 19, 819, 1977.
4. Kerr, P. S., Recording occupational health data for future analysis, *J. Occup. Med.*, 20, 197, 1978.
5. Pell, S., Epidemiological requirements for medical-environmental data management, *J. Occup. Med.*, 20, 554, 1978.
6. Pell, S., O'Berg, M. T., and Karrh, B. W., Cancer epidemiologic surveillance in the Du Pont Company, *J. Occup. Med.*, 20, 725, 1978.
7. Department of Labor, Occupational Safety and Health Administration, Identification, classification, and regulation of toxic substances posing a potential occupational carcinogenic risk, *Fed. Regist.*, 42, 54148, 1977.
8. Eighth International Classification of Disease, PHS Publ. No. 1693, U.S. Department of Health, Education and Welfare, Washington, D.C., 1967.
9. Cole, P. and Morrison, A. S., Basic issues in population screening for cancer, *J. Nat. Cancer Inst.*, in press.
10. Monson, R. R., Foster, L., Louik, C., and Peters, J. M., Morbidity survey — B. F. Goodrich Company, unpubl. rep., Dec. 15, 1976.
11. Sparks, P., Monson, R. R., and Andjelkovich, D., Effects upon the developing fetus of parental employment in the rubber industry, 1980, in progress.

12. American Medical Association, *Standard Nomenclature of Diseases and Operations,* 5th ed., Thompson, E. T., and Hayden, A. C., Eds., McGraw-Hill, New York, 1961.

13. **Slone, D., Shapiro, S., and Miettinen, O. S.,** Case-control surveillance of serious illnesses attributable to ambulatory drug use, in *Epidemiological Evaluation of Drugs,* Columbo, F., Shapiro, S., Slone, D., and Tognoni, G., Eds., Elsevier, Amsterdam, 1977, 59.

14. **Slone, D., Shapiro, S., Rosenberg, L., Kaufman, D. W., Hartz, S. C. Rossi, A. C., Stolley, P. D., and Miettinen, O. S.,** Relation of cigarette smoking to myocardial infarction in young women, *N. Engl. J. Med.,* 298, 1273, 1978.

Chapter 9
CURRENT PROBLEMS IN OCCUPATIONAL EPIDEMIOLOGY

I. INTRODUCTION

The purpose of occupational epidemiology is to provide information on human health that can be used to prevent human illness. As time goes by data accumulate on the relationship between occupational exposures and human diseases. Some of these data can be interpreted unequivocally and can provide a firm basis for a change in behavior. Other data are subject to more than one interpretation or may be challenged as to veracity. As indicated throughout these pages, data by themselves provide no indication as to whether or not they reflect true processes in human populations.

In this chapter a variety of problems related to occupational exposures are considered. These problems are illustrated by referring to recent literature in occupational epidemiology. The intent is to provide an overview of general problems rather than to provide a detailed review of specific issues. Excellent reviews of the known and suspected effects of exposure to substances used in industry can be found in the Criteria Documents published by the National Institute for Occupational Safety and Health (NIOSH) and in the reports of the International Agency for Research in Cancer (IARC).[1,2]

For each of the studies reviewed in this chapter, the collection, analysis, and interpretation of the data are presented and the meaning of the results is discussed. Some of the studies are models on how to conduct research; some of the studies illustrate problems in methodology that should be avoided. All of the studies illustrate the realities encountered in conducting research in occupational epidemiology and in interpreting the results of that research.

II. OCCUPATION AND REPRODUCTIVE EFFECTS

Exposure to substances used in industry may lead to effects on the reproductive system in men or in women or may lead to an effect on the unborn fetus. Few data have been published on the general relationship between occupation and problems of reproduction. Until recently few pregnant women have been exposed to industrial environments. Any effects on male workers are difficult to detect. Any effects on fetuses have not been studied to any extent.

A. Vinyl Chloride and Fetal Deaths

In October 1974, interviews were conducted with male workers exposed to vinyl chloride monomer (VCM), polyvinyl-chloride (PVC) or rubber.[3] Questions were asked about the interviewee's health as well as about the outcomes of pregnancy of the workers' wives. The fetal death rate subsequent to exposure for VCM was higher among the families of exposed men than among the families of controls (Table 9.1).

This study is difficult to classify. It is not a retrospective cohort study, because workers were not followed either in retrospect or in prospect for the occurrence of fetal deaths. It is not a case-control study, because subject selection was not based on presence or absence of fetal deaths. It is best thought of as a cross-sectional study where exposure is presence or absence of a history of VCM exposure and disease is presence or absence of having had fetal death. A potential problem is that there may have been a differential rate of termination of employment according to exposure-disease status. The data seen in Table 9.1 could result if exposure to VCM did not

Table 9.1
FETAL DEATH RATES AMONG FAMILIES OF
MEN EXPOSED TO VINYL CHLORIDE
MONOMER AND AMONG FAMILIES OF
CONTROLS

| | Fetal death rate[a] | | | |
| | Prior to exposure | | Subsequent to exposure | |
Group	Crude	Standardized	Crude	Standardized
Exposed	10.1	6.1	16.5	15.8
Controls	6.9	6.9	8.8	8.8

[a]   Number of fetal deaths per 100 pregnancies.

lead to increased fetal death, but if controls with fetal deaths terminated at a higher rate than exposed workers with fetal deaths. This can be thought of as selection bias.

Selection bias also was possible because not all workers eligible for the study were interviewed. The data in Table 9.1 could have resulted if exposed workers with a history of fetal deaths selectively agreed to participate in the study.

Because the interviews were not conducted blindly, observation bias was possible. The data in Table 9.1 could result if workers with exposure to VCM over-reported, or if controls under-reported, the occurrence of fetal deaths.

No information on smoking of mothers is presented. Smoking is known to be associated with an increased fetal death rate.[4] The data in Table 9.1 could have resulted from confounding by smoking if the wives of VCM workers smoked more than the wives of controls.

The primary procedure used in the analysis was direct standardization of rates, because the age distribution differed between exposed and control groups. Because the standard used was the age-distribution of the controls, the crude and standardized rates for controls in Table 9.1 were identical. For the exposed, there was a substantial reduction in the standardized rate prior to exposure. This occurred because the exposed group was older than the control group, and because the rate of fetal deaths increased with age (Table 9.2).[5]

In this example the standardization behaved well, since the age-standardized rates as well as the age-specific rates showed essentially no differences in fetal death rates between the exposed and the control groups. However, the potential difficulties of direct standardization with respect to small numbers can be seen. If there had been more controls in the <20 category, and if there had been two or three fetal deaths among the seven exposed persons in the <20 category, that stratum would have contributed heavily to a high standardized rate among the exposed group. In such a situation, it is best to limit the analysis to overlapping age-strata in which there are sufficient numbers, e.g., ages 20 to 29. In any standardization procedure attention must be given to the elements being standardized.

The meaning of this single study is unclear. Some of the criticisms raised above must be viewed as far-fetched. The likelihood of selection bias seems remote. The possibility of observation bias is more real, inasmuch as the interviews were conducted shortly after the carcinogenic properties of vinyl chloride were announced. If anything, the fetal death rate of 8.8% in controls seems low, suggesting that they may have not been stimulated sufficiently to recall previous miscarriages in their wives. It seems unlikely that the smoking habits of the wives of these two groups of workers would differ; even

Table 9.2

FETAL DEATH RATES PRIOR TO EXPOSURE AMONG FAMILIES
OF MEN EXPOSED TO VINYL CHLORIDE MONOMER AND
AMONG CONTROLS ACCORDING TO AGE OF FATHER

		Age of father					
	Group	<20	20—24	25—29	30—34	≥35	All
Number of pregnancies	Exposed	7	44	56	27	14	148
	Control	31	80	38	6	4	159
Fetal death rate[a]	Exposed	0.0	4.5	12.5	18.5	7.1	10.1
	Control	6.5	5.0	10.5	16.7	0.0	6.9

[a] Number of fetal deaths per 100 pregnancies.

if wives of exposed men smoked more, the association between smoking and fetal deaths is weaker than the association seen in this study.

As suggested by the above paragraph, the meaning of the results of this study is a matter of opinion, not of science. Different persons will raise different criticisms or different defenses. Certainly the results of this one study are not definitive.

With respect to future public health policy, it is not a major concern whether vinyl chloride exposure to men tends to increased fetal deaths among their offspring. The association between VCM and angiosarcoma is many times stronger and therefore VCM exposure must be reduced. Such reduction would be expected to minimize any adverse effects of VCM on the reproductive system.

However, it is of public health concern that VCM might affect pregnant women directly. In order to address this concern, studies must be made of pregnant women exposed to VCM and of their children.

B. Paternal Occupation and Childhood Cancer

1. Children in Quebec

"In reviewing, for other purposes, a small sample of birth and death certificates of Quebec children, the impression emerged of a large number of fathers in petrol-related occupations when the cause of death was cancer."[6] To quantify this impression, the occupation of the father was obtained from the birth certificate of 386 children under the age of 5 who died from cancer. For comparison purposes, two matched controls per case were selected — the preceding and succeeding child in the birth certificate registry. As seen in Table 9.3, approximately twice as many cases had fathers with potential exposure to petrol and other hydrocarbons. The odds ratio is $(71 \times 697) \div (75 \times 315) = 2.1$. The 95% confidence interval of the odds ratio is 1.5 to 3.0.

Selection bias is an unlikely explanation since paternal occupation was not ascertained until after cases were defined. Observation bias could have led to these results. The authors admit to a prior notion that petro-related occupations were related to childhood cancer. In classifying a father's occupation, it is possible that occupations difficult to classify were coded as petrol-related for cases but not for controls. However, the authors state that occupation was coded by a person who was blinded as to case-control status. Thus, for this reason, observation bias was not possible.

Confounding by some factor related to occupation and childhood cancer could always be an explanation. However, no data on potential confounding factors were available from the birth certificate, except for age. The mean paternal age for both cases and controls was 31.4. Further, little is known as to determinants of childhood cancer.

Table 9.3

OCCUPATION OF FATHER AT TIME OF BIRTH AMONG
CHILDREN DYING OF CANCER IN QUEBEC AND AMONG
CONTROL CHILDREN

Occupation of father	Children with cancer	Control children
Motor-vehicle mechanic	28	27
Machinist	24	29
Other hydrocarbon exposure	19	19
Other	315	697
Total	386	772

Odds ratio = 2.1

The data can be criticzed if they include the cases upon whom the initial impression was based. It may be that the initial impression was correct, but was based on a sample of children with cancer who were simply atypical because of chance. In order to test the correctness of the impression, independent data should be evaluated. It is not stated in this report whether or not this was done.

In the analysis of data a large number of occupations were coded. The data in Table 9.3 are derived from a much larger Table. The association with hydrocarbon-related occupations is partially a result of looking through a number of occupations and grouping those which appear to be related to hydrocarbon exposure. However, this grouping seems to have been done without regard for disease status; for example, among the "other hydrocarbon exposure" grouping were three cleaners among controls and only one among cases.

A criticism might be made that a matched analysis was not done. However, if the controls were matched to cases for purposes of control of confounding, the lack of a matched analysis would only dilute any association between exposure and disease. The occurrence of an odds ratio of 2.1 (instead of 1.0) could not be attributed to the non-matched nature of the analysis. Further, the matching was done essentially for purposes of convenience rather than of control of confounding. A matched analysis was not called for.

It is difficult to interpret the results of a single study such as this. While the association is probably real in this population at this time, it is not necessarily causal. The fact that the association is statistically significant does not mean that it could not have occurred by chance. The only change in behavior dictated by this study should be to collect further data.

2. Children in Finland

In response to the above study, an analysis was done of data collected in a Finnish study of childhood cancer. Cases were children under the age of 15 who developed, rather than died from, cancer. One control for each case was selected; the control was the child born immediately before the case in the same maternity welfare district. Paternal occupation was routinely recorded for all children at the first visit of the mother to the maternity welfare center. As seen in Table 9.4, there was no association of paternal hydrocarbon exposure with childhood cancer. The 95% confidence limits of the odds ratio of 1.0 were 0.8 and 1.3.

The data in this study indicate no association between paternal hydrocarbon exposure and childhood cancer. Criticisms must be directed at factors that may have led to the failure to detect a true association, should one have existed.

Table 9.4
OCCUPATION OF FATHER AT TIME OF CONCEPTION AMONG CHILDREN DEVELOPING CANCER IN FINLAND AND AMONG CONTROL CHILDREN

Occupation of father	Children with cancer	Controls
Hydrocarbon exposure	109	109
Other	743	743
Total	852	852

Odds ratio = 1.0

Random misclassification must be considered. With respect to disease, little misclassification is likely. Few children with the diagnosis of cancer do not have the disease; few children without the diagnosis have latent disease. However, the determination of petrol exposure in the father is not a precise procedure. It is possible that some fathers said not to have exposure in fact did and vice versa. However, in order for an odds ratio of 1.0 to result from random misclassification, there would have to be no relationship between true paternal occupation and classified paternal occupation. This seems unlikely.

Selection bias could have led to these results, assuming that paternal exposure to hydrocarbons led to childhood cancer, only through a rather convoluted process. Cases who had fathers with hydrocarbon exposure would have had to be selectively excluded from the study or controls who had fathers with hydrocarbon exposure would have had to be selectively included. Inasmuch as the data were collected prior to any hypothesis as to hydrocarbon exposure of childhood cancer, this possibility seems remote. For the same reason, there seems to be little likelihood that paternal occupation was ascertained differently from cases and controls.

In order for confounding bias to have led to data in which there was no association between exposure and disease, negative confounding must have occurred. Some factor that was a cause of childhood cancer would have had to be more common among the controls than among the cases. Since little is known as to the causes of childhood cancer, such a factor would be difficult to identify. There is known to be a weak association between prenatal X-ray and childhood cancer.[8] If there were more X-rayed children among fathers with *no* hydrocarbon exposure, negative confounding would be possible. However, the association between childhood cancer and prenatal X-ray is very weak (OR $\sim$ 1.5) and could not mask a true odds ratio of 2.1.

3. Comment

These two studies led to data that are not compatible on statistical grounds. The 95% confidence limits do not overlap and thus it is quite unlikely that results such as these would result simply because of random variation in the selection of two samples from the same universe. However, the data from these studies are not at all atypical of data collected in the epidemiologic setting. It is relatively common for two studies to lead to grossly different results that do not seem to be explainable for methodologic reasons.

Whenever an association is first reported, as in the Quebec study, it is reasonable to report the association and to comment briefly on the possible meaning. If there is broad general truth to the association, this will be quickly recognized and substantiating data will soon be assembled. There is no need for the authors either to defend their data against detractors or to announce their wide generalizability. The authors of the Quebec study behaved in a proper conservative manner by recommending only that further investigation be done.

When the results in Quebec became known, persons with interest in the general problem considered how to examine further the relationship between paternal hydrocarbon exposure and childhood cancer. Among these persons were those who believed that the association was causal, those who believed that the association was nonsense, and those who were agnostic. Each type of person considered the possibility of collecting further data: some may have wanted to collect confirmatory data, some may have wanted to collect contradictory data, and some wanted simply to collect data. There is no necessary connection between a person's opinion as to the truth of some association and his desire to collect data that confirms or refutes the association. However, it might be supposed that there will be a tendency for true believers to collect contradictory data. Agnostics will not necessarily collect true data, for their seeming neutrality may only be a mask covering some hidden bias.

The first data to appear after the initial report of some association tend to be the result of expedience rather than of a desire to confirm or refute the association. The Finland paper resulted from an analysis of data collected for another reason and presumably free of bias. Had this paper been authored by representatives of the oil industry, there would be a natural reaction that the industry was out to cover-up the harmful effects of paternal occupation. However, if a confirmatory paper had been published by representatives of the oil industry there would be a strong desire on the part of the general scientific community to believe the causal nature of the association.

As time passes, other data will appear on the relationship between paternal exposure to hydrocarbons and childhood cancer. One might expect that data that show no association will be viewed as being "uninteresting" and will not be published, while data that show an association will be published. These are emotional human responses to data. However, it seems unlikely that there is a strong tendency in science for such preferential publication of data that show association. As in this situation, whenever a positive study appears, a negative study frequently follows.

The judgment as to the ultimate truth as to whether the exposure causes the disease is not a matter of adding up the positive and the negative studies. Each study must be considered as to its merits. It is possible that all studies are correct; the exposure may cause the disease in one population but not in others. It is not necessary that universal truth be the final result of the consideration of the results of a number of scientific studies.

With respect to the specific association between paternal hydrocarbon exposure and childhood cancer, the question is still undecided. There is no obvious reason to fault one or the other study. While on general principles it would be wise to limit exposure to hydrocarbons, there is as yet no need to set a specific standard of exposure because of likely damage to the future children of a man exposed to petrol.

C. Summary

Much work is needed in general on the etiology of birth defects and specifically on the possible role of occupation. I believe that epidemiologic surveillance systems on industrial populations are ideally suited to such study. The outcome of birth occurs close in time to the exposure; a number of medical visits and insurance payments take place during a pregnancy and delivery; any abnormality of the child usually is apparent at or shortly after birth.

Epidemiologic surveillance systems on industrial populations should be designed so as to incorporate data on pregnancies among wives of male workers. At the preemployment history, information may be obtained as to previous reproductive history. If pregnancy expenses are paid by a company-supported insurance program, data on the pregnancy and its outcome should be readily available from the insurance company and/or the hospital.

Because any adverse outcomes of pregnancy related to work are likely to be of relatively low frequency, large amounts of data will be necessary to detect any association. Therefore, it seems reasonable that groups of companies within specific industries pool their data or share their findings. Much of the data collected will be routine and of little interpretive value. However, if an abnormality of pregnancy is caused by some parental work exposure, it should be detected as soon as possible. Elimination of the responsible substance has the potential to lead in a relatively short time to elimination of the adverse health effect. This contrasts with the years or decades needed to demonstrate the successful elimination of an occupational carcinogen.

III. OCCUPATION AND RESPIRATORY CANCER

Currently, there is concern over the role of chemicals in the etiology of cancer. It is hypothesized that long-term low-level exposure to environmental pollutants may be responsible for a high percentage of cancer.[9] However, it is difficult to study this question in the general population; no records exist on past exposures to these pollutants and doing prospective cohort studies would be expensive and of questionable feasibility. Persons working in industry are exposed to higher levels of many chemicals; some rough estimate can usually be obtained as to past exposure; the conduct of retrospective cohort studies on industrial populations is relatively inexpensive and feasible. Therefore, much can be learned about the role of chemicals in the development of human cancer by studying industrial populations.

There is a wide spectrum of current knowledge as to the relationship between industrial exposure to chemicals and cancer. For some substances there is an unquestioned relationship between a substance and a cancer; standards of exposure to the substance exist, are enforced and seem to be effective. For some industrial settings there is agreement that the general exposure is harmful even though there is no specific association between a substance and a disease. Standards in the setting are aimed at general environment rather than specific exposure. In other settings there is a contested association between exposure and disease; to some observers an association represents cause and effect while to others the association is an example of bias. Finally, there are situations in which the data are conflicting and most agree that no conclusions are possible at the moment.

In this section the relationship between occupation and respiratory cancer is considered. For some occupational exposures, there is a clear-cut causal association with respiratory cancer. For other exposures, excess respiratory cancer has been reported but disagreement exists as to whether the association is causal.

A. Nickel and Respiratory Cancer

In 1949 on the basis of clinical reports, cancers of the nose or lung among workers exposed to nickel were classified as industrial diseases.[10] To quantify this association, a study was done of the occupation of 15,247 men who died from lung cancer, from nasal cancer, or from other causes.[10] This study was done of deaths between 1938 and 1956 in an area of Great Britain where a nickel refinery was located.

The data were collected by a review of death certificates. Cause of death was coded in accordance with standard procedures; the occupation of each decedent was that listed on the death certificate. The relationship between cause of death and occupation is given in Table 9.5. Excesses of nasal cancer and of lung cancer among decedents in the nickel industry are apparent.

It is difficult to construct a realistic argument that the associations seen in Table 9.5 are the result of bias. All deaths of men residing in this area were included; therefore there was no selection. Selection bias could have resulted if men who were employed in the nickel industry and who died from "other causes" migrated from Great Britain before death, but this seems unlikely. There is also no reason to believe that nasal and lung cancers were over-certified as the cause of death in men who worked in the nickel industry. Confounding by cigarette smoking could be considered for the excess of lung cancer, but is extremely unlikely. In those years a very high proportion of British males smoked; therefore even if nickel workers smoked more than other workers, the amount of confounding possible was minimal. Cigarette smoking has little, if any, effect on nasal cancer.

A question can be raised as to the basic study design and the way the data were analyzed. The data were based solely on death certificates. No follow-up was made of a group of nickel workers and no mortality rates were available. The study was essentially a proportional mortality study in which the percentage of nasal and lung cancers were compared among various groups of workers.

Crudely, the proportion of nasal cancer among nickel workers was 0.065 [13/(13 + 48 + 139)]. Among "other" employees the proportion was 0.00064 and among all employees the proportion was 0.0016. The ratio of the proportion of cancer among nickel workers to the proportion among "other" employees was 100:1. If the ratio is computed relative to the "total" group, it is 40:1. Irrespective of which group is used for comparison, the excess nasal cancer among nickel workers is apparent. The proportion of lung cancer among nickel workers (0.24) was also substantially higher than the proportion among "other" workers (0.05).

Because of the strong association between employment in the nickel industries and cancers of the nasal sinuses and lung, the study design and analysis could be simple. The error introduced by the use of proportional mortality is perhaps 10 to 30%; the error introduced from the lack of age-standardization is also small. These errors can have little effect on the 4000% excess of nasal cancer or the 500% excess of lung cancer among nickel workers. The causal nature of the association can readily be accepted.

However, the determination of a safe level of exposure to workers in nickel refineries is much more difficult. Safety cannot be considered to be achieved until no excess nasal or lung cancers occur. For nasal cancer, because of its rarity, this means no cases must occur among nickel workers. For lung cancer, which is largely determined by cigarette smoking habits, some nonzero number must be expected among any group of persons who smoke.

In 1970, the occurrence of deaths among a cohort of nickel workers was reported.[11] Eight hundred and forty-five men who had been employed in a nickel refinery in South Wales were followed from 1939 through 1966. Excess nasal cancer among nickel workers was suspected in 1927 and the refining process was changed between 1925 and 1933.[11, 12] Therefore, it was of particular interest to determine whether any excess nasal or lung cancer had occurred in men first exposed after 1925.

Because this was a retrospective cohort study, the observed number of deaths could be compared to the number expected based on national death rates. The results are presented in Table 9.6. No nasal cancer occurred in men who were first employed after 1924; only a slight excess of lung cancer was seen in these men. It might be concluded that the change in process led to the prevention of nickel-induced cancer.

However, in 1977 an updated follow-up was presented (Table 9.7).[12] Among men

Table 9.5
CAUSE OF DEATH AMONG PERSONS EMPLOYED IN NICKEL AND IN OTHER INDUSTRIES IN GREAT BRITAIN

Industry of employment	Cause of death		
	Nasal cancer	Lung cancer	Other causes
Nickel	13	48	139
Other Refining	1	54	606
Steel	3	121	2,055
Coal-mining	2	73	2,729
Other	6	503	8,894
Total	25	799	14,423

Table 9.6
OBSERVED/EXPECTED CAUSES OF DEATH AMONG NICKEL WORKERS ACCORDING TO YEAR OF FIRST EMPLOYMENT; FOLLOW-UP 1939 to 1966

Year of first employment	Cause of death		
	Nasal cancer	Lung cancer	Other causes
<1925	39/0.11	105/13.9	263/208.7
1925—29	0/0.01	4/2.3	23/23.7
1930—44	0/0.02	4/3.8	44/33.9

who started employment between 1925 and 1929, one case of nasal cancer occurred. An excess of lung cancer was seen in both groups of men who were first employed after 1925. While this excess is relatively much smaller than that observed in men who started working before 1925, it suggests that some workers employed after 1924 developed lung cancer because of their work.

In this example, data on men who started working between 1925 and 1929 are being evaluated in 1977 to determine whether or not nickel workers develop excess cancer. It might be assumed that the risks to workers of today will be no higher than the risks to the workers in 1925. However, it seems clear that one cannot conclude that the changes instituted in nickel refining around 1925 were sufficient to prevent the development of work-related nasal or lung cancer.

The specific agent responsible for the excess cancers is not known. While both nickel and nickel carbonyl gas are carcinogenic,[13] excess nasal and lung cancer has also been observed in men exposed mainly to nickel ore dusts.[14] Had controls been instituted in 1925 only against elemental nickel and nickel carbonyl gas, the reduction in excess respiratory cancer might have been much less.

A parallel to the nickel cancers may be seen in vinyl chloride. The excess occurrence of a rare cancer (angiosarcoma of the liver) was recognized on clinical grounds.[15] Clinical recognition was possible because the disease had few other causes and had a very high rate ratio associated with the exposure (100 +). The process of producing vinyl chloride has been changed so that exposure is greatly reduced.[16] However, it is unknown as to whether these controls will prevent the occurrence of angiosarcoma.

Also, the possible excess occurrence of cancers of the lung and of the brain among

Table 9.7

OBSERVED/EXPECTED CAUSES OF DEATH AMONG
NICKEL WORKERS ACCORDING TO YEAR OF FIRST
EMPLOYMENT; FOLLOW-UP 1934 TO 1971

	Cause of death		
Year of first employment	Nasal cancer	Lung cancer	Other causes
<1925	56/0.17	128/18.4	368/378.0
1925—29	0/0.03[a]	9/3.6	51/48.3
1930—44	0/0.03	8/5.5	69/54.9

[a]　One man developed nasal cancer but died from heart disease.

workers exposed to vinyl chloride have been reported in a proportional mortality study.[17] If vinyl chloride leads to these cancers, the rate ratio is many times less than that for angiosarcoma. Further, these cancers are much more frequent among the general population and might be expected to occur among vinyl chloride workers for non-causal reasons. It may be difficult to demonstrate that the occurrence of one of these diseases in a vinyl chloride worker is not due to vinyl chloride exposure.

Also, it should be clear that at the moment the decision as to the "safe" level of exposure to vinyl chloride is a matter of opinion rather than of science. In one study no excess cases of angiosarcoma, lung cancer, or brain cancer were reported.[18] It is possible that workers at this plant were exposed to safe levels of vinyl chloride. However, it is also possible that insufficient time has passed for any vinyl chloride-induced cancer to develop. The setting of a standard of exposure to vinyl chloride had to be based on a process of negotiation between government and industry. The standard must be conservative, i.e., because of the uncertainty associated with what is a safe level of vinyl chloride, the standard should, if anything, be too low.

B. Coke Ovens and Respiratory Cancer*

In 1962, a collaborative study of the mortality experience of steelworkers was initiated by the U.S. Public Health Service, the Graduate School of Public Health of the University of Pittsburgh, and three large steel companies.[20] The purpose of the study was to assess conflicting reports of excess illness among certain groups of steelworkers.

As of 1953, there were 59,072 men employed in seven steel plants in Allegheny County, Pennsylvania. In 1962—64 an attempt was made to determine the vital status as of 1/1/62 of each of these men. There were 32,263 men who were still employed, 6346 who had retired, but were alive, 15,650 who had left employment but were alive, and 4716 who were deceased. Only 97 men could not be located.

As seen in Table 9.8, the observed mortality among this group was 82% of that expected on the basis of Allegheny County rates. Among all steelworkers, there was no overall excess of cancer.

The next step was to break down the study group of steelworkers according to their usual area of employment.[21] So as to minimize the difficulties associated with persons changing jobs, an analysis was done including a man in a given work area only if he worked there for at least 5 years. In order to eliminate the over-estimation of expected deaths, the death rates of men who worked in each work area for at least 5 years were

* This section is taken from a paper in a symposium on the environment in *Environmental Law*.[19] See also Chapter 3.

Table 9.8
OBSERVED AND EXPECTED
DEATHS AMONG STEELWORKERS[a]

Cause of death	Observed	Expected	SMR[b]
All causes	4716	5766.8	82
All cancer	1008	1091.4	92
CNS vascular	365	464.3	79
Heart disease	1906	2311.3	82
External	474	450.5	105
All other causes	963	1449.3	66

[a] Expected numbers based on mortality rates for Allegheny County, Pennsylvania.
[b] SMR = Standardized mortality ratio = 100 × observed/expected.

Table 9.9
OBSERVED AND EXPECTED DEATHS FOR ALL
CAUSES AND ALL CANCERS AMONG
STEELWORKERS EMPLOYED AT LEAST FIVE
YEARS IN SPECIFIED WORK AREAS[a]

Work area	Race	All causes		All cancer	
		Obs.	Exp.	Obs.	Exp.
Coke plant	White	130	130.8	29	28.3
	Non-white	96	78.7	40	19.6
Cold reducing mills	White	71	70.7	17	14.6
	Non-white	14	6.3	1	1.4
General labor	White	102	81.6	16	18.4
	Non-white	49	46.1	14	11.4
Maintenance	White	377	318.4	76	70.1
	Non-white	16	14.3	3	3.8
Merchant mills	White	253	266.9	65	59.1
	Non-white	28	42.4	5	10.7

[a] Expected numbers based on mortality rates for all steelworkers who worked at least 5 years.

compared to the rates of all steelworkers in the study who worked at least 5 years. The results of this analysis are presented in Table 9.9.

Among all causes of death, no "healthy worker effect" is seen, since the mortality rate used for comparison was that of all steelworkers rather than that of a general population. Moderate excesses of death are seen among nonwhite workers in the coke plant and the cold reducing mills and among white workers in the general labor and maintenance areas. With respect to all cancer, however, a striking excess is seen among nonwhite workers in the coke plant. Most of this excess was found to be due to lung cancer.

Several questions were raised by this finding:

1.   Why was there a difference in the ratio of observed to expected deaths between whites and nonwhites who had worked at least 5 years at the coke plant?
2.   Did nonwhite coke area workers smoke cigarettes more than other steelworkers?
3.   Could this excess reflect a causal association between working in the coke plant and lung cancer? If so, was there evidence that whites and nonwhites had different jobs?
4.   What exposures were present in the coke plant?

In the coke plant, coal was heated under reduced concentration of oxygen so as to produce coke. Coke is used in the smelting of steel. In the heating of the coal, many chemicals are volatilized and released into the air. While much of this volatilized chemical fume is collected, some is not. Further, when the ovens are opened to remove the red-hot coke and to refill the oven with coal, much of the fume is released. Men whose job it is to remove coke and add coal have continual exposure to the by-products of the process.

At this stage, the reason for the excess lung cancer among nonwhite coke plant workers was not clear. It could reflect the confounding effects of cigarette smoking or other factors, it could reflect a causal association, or it could simply be due to chance. It must be emphasized that chance can never be ruled out as a reason for an association. It may be judged to be extremely unlikely, but never absolutely impossible.

While the tentative judgment was that this was a causal association, it was felt that further information should be collected. The steelworkers were followed for five additional years and employment status prior to 1953 was considered. Among men who had worked at least 5 years in the coke plant, a distinction was made between oven and nonoven workers. The nonoven workers had relatively clean jobs not directly connected with the making of coke.[22]

The results are presented in Table 9.10. Relative to all steelworkers, there is about a 10% excess of death from all causes in each group. Among workers in the oven area, there is almost an 80% excess of all cancer; an excess of approximately 25% is seen among nonoven workers. The excess among coke oven workers is primarily due to lung cancer. Also, there is a 400% excess of kidney cancer. Among nonoven workers, there is a deficit of lung cancer. However, there is an excess of death due to digestive cancer.

The data in Tables 9.9 and 9.10 are assumed to represent a causal association between working at the coke oven and lung cancer. Nonwhites tend to work in the oven area and whites tend to work in the nonoven area. There is no evidence that nonwhite oven workers smoked cigarettes to excess. The atmosphere around the coke oven contains a mixture of chemicals present in coal. Many of these chemicals are known to be carcinogenic in animals. It makes good sense that these chemicals are inhaled by persons working in the oven area and with time cause lung cancer.

However, other excesses are present in Table 9.10. Do these represent causal associations? The answer is not clear-cut. For example, there is an excess of kidney cancer in each group. While this is based on a small absolute number of deaths, the relative excess (6/1.5) is large. Also, there is an excess of digestive cancer among nonoven workers. In contrast to lung cancer, little is known about the causes of these cancers. There have been reports of excesses of various types of digestive cancers among other groups of workers, but there is no obvious relation between the working conditions in those jobs and coke plant jobs.

Based on the data in this study, a coke oven standard has been established.[23] Respiratory protection is required for the men who work at the oven. This seems reasonable in light of the excess lung cancer. But what if the only excesses seen had been kidney

Table 9.10

OBSERVED AND EXPECTED
DEATHS AMONG STEELWORKERS
EMPLOYED IN THE COKE PLANT
FOR AT LEAST 5 YEARS PRIOR TO
1953[a]

Cause of death	Coke oven		Nonoven	
	Obs.	Exp.	Obs.	Exp.
All causes	214	192.4	178	163.5
All cancer	75	43.9	43	34.6
Lung	40	14.1	5	9.7
Digestive	14	13.9	20	12.6
Kidney	4	0.8	2	0.7
CNS vascular	20	18.6	20	14.6
Heart	56	70.5	77	72.4
Accidents	11	9.4	8	6.6
All other causes	52	50.0	30	35.3

[a] Expected numbers based on mortality rates for
all steelworkers who worked at least 5 years.

and digestive cancers? The judgment as to the causal nature of the associations would have been less clear and the need for protection of the worker less obvious. While it is logical to argue for increased worker protection whenever a health risk is suspected, the nature of the protection and the cost required to provide the protection must be considered. Management is reluctant to provide costly protective measures when there is little or no evidence that such protection will in fact be of benefit. Since there usually is room for disagreement as to what constitutes a health risk, there will always be a need for an impartial review of the evidence.

Several points are to be made on the steelworker experience:

1. The expected number of deaths for specific causes differs depending upon the comparison population being used. In this study some comparisons involved all steelworkers vs. the Allegheny County general populations. Others involved a subgroup of steelworkers. Other comparisons might have been done, e.g., all steelworkers vs. the U.S. general population or coke plant workers vs. general laborers vs. maintenance workers. Each of these comparisons will usually produce a different expected number of deaths. Therefore, interpretation of data from any one comparison must be cautious. The possibility must be kept in mind that other comparisons will yield different, and possibly more accurate, results.

2. The causal nature of coke oven work with lung cancer was not immediately obvious to everyone. Since cigarette smoking is known to cause most of the lung cancer in the general population, the possible confounding effects of smoking had to be considered.

3. Amplification of the original findings was necessary. Further analysis of the initial data to separate exposure led to a more specific association of job and disease.

4. The knowledge as to the magnitude of the association between coke oven work and lung cancer is imprecise. Consequently, the only approach to prevention must be based on respiratory protection aimed at eliminating exposure to coke oven fumes.

Table 9.11
OBSERVED AND EXPECTED DEATHS FROM LUNG CANCER AMONG A COHORT OF 17,800 ASBESTOS INSULATION WORKERS

Cigarette smoking habit	No. of persons	Deaths from lung cancer			
		1967—1972		1967—1975	
		Obs.	Exp.[a]	Obs.	Exp.[b]
Yes	9590	179	31.6	248	59.5
No	2066	2	7.5	6	2.3
Unknown	6144	94	16.8	—	—

[a] Expected numbers based on age-specific U.S. death rates for white males.

[b] Expected numbers based on approximate age-smoking specific U.S. death rates for white males.

5.   The nature of the association between coke plant work and kidney cancer and nonoven work and digestive cancer is unclear. However, it is possible that providing respiratory protection to reduce the occurrence of lung cancer will also reduce the occurrence of other diseases.

C. Asbestos and Respiratory Cancer

There is no question that persons who work with asbestos develop excess respiratory cancer.[24] There is a question, however, as to whether asbestos exposure in the absence of cigarette smoking will lead to an excess of lung cancer. This question has recently been reviewed.[25]

In 1967, smoking habits were ascertained from 11,656 of 17,800 insulation workers who were exposed to asbestos. These workers have been followed since that time and deaths from lung cancer have been determined. In one analysis, expected numbers of deaths from lung cancer were estimated on the basis of U.S. death rates of smokers and nonsmokers combined.[26] In a second analysis, estimated rates for smokers and nonsmokers were used to compute expected numbers.[27]

The results of these two analyses are presented in Table 9.11. In the first analysis (1967 to 1972) there is no evidence that absestos exposure in the absence of cigarette smoking leads to an excess of lung cancer. This statement, however, must be tempered by the high number of persons with an unknown smoking habit. The observed/expected ratio in these persons is essentially the same as that among the smokers. It is conceivable that a number of the persons with lung cancer among those whose smoking habits are unknown were nonsmokers. The true observed/expected ratio among nonsmokers could be above 1.0.

Another objection to these data can be raised concerning the rates upon which the expected numbers were based. Vital statistics rates are not available for smokers and nonsmokers separately. (It would be almost impossible to collect such data from the general population.) Therefore, expected numbers must be computed on the basis of the general population, which is a mixture of smokers and nonsmokers. As a result, the expected numbers of lung cancer for smokers are underestimated while the expected numbers for nonsmokers are overestimated. In the second analysis of the data,[27] an estimated smoking-specific lung cancer mortality rate was used to compute expected numbers.[24] Also, in this analysis three additional years had passed; therefore the observed number of deaths from lung cancer had increased. It can be seen in the 1967-

Table 9.12
ASSOCIATION BETWEEN LUNG CANCER AND SHIP BUILDING ACCORDING TO SMOKING IN A CASE-CONTROL STUDY

Cigarette smoking habit	Shipbuilder	Lung cancer Yes	Lung cancer No	Odds ratio
No or light	Yes	11	35	1.3
	No	50	203	
Moderate	Yes	70	42	1.7
	No	217	220	
Heavy	Yes	14	3	2.4
	No	96	50	

75 data in Table 11 that there is a suggestion that nonsmoking asbestos insulation workers also had an excess of lung cancer.

The question as to the interrelationship between asbestos, cigarette smoking, and lung cancer has also been examined in a case-control study.[28] In an examination of the cancer maps by U.S. County in 1950 to 69, an excess of lung cancer was observed among white males.[29] To evaluate the reason for this excess, a case-control study of lung cancer was conducted among residents of coastal Georgia. Cases were men with lung cancer identified during several periods since 1970; controls were persons with other diseases identified either from hospital records or from death certificates. Persons with bladder cancer or chronic lung disease were not eligible to be controls, inasmuch as these diseases are known to occur to excess among cigarette smokers. Controls were matched to cases on sex, race, age, county of residence, and vital statistics.

Interviews were conducted with living cases and controls and with the next-of-kin of persons who were deceased. Information was obtained as to past smoking habits and occupational histories. At the conclusion of the interview, specific questions were asked about ship building and asbestos exposure. During World War II, ship building, which involves asbestos exposure, was common in this area.

The results are presented in Table 9.12. Among non or light smokers, the odds ratio of lung cancer in ship builders was 1.3, while among heavy smokers, the odds ratio was 2.4. While the association between lung cancer and ship building, and presumably asbestos, is much weaker than that seen among insulation workers, it is in the same direction.

The major concern to be considered in this study is in the way the data were collected. The study was done to evaluate the role of ship building in the etiology of lung cancer. Consequently, it was very important to phrase questions to the persons in the study in a neutral way, so as to avoid observation bias in the collection of occupational histories. Since the shipyards had operated for only a few years during World War II, and since the occupational histories were obtained by interview in the mid-1970s, it was possible that incomplete occupational histories might be given. If this incompleteness occurred equally among cases and controls, no bias would result. However, if cases were prompted more than controls as to past work in a shipyard, a false association between shipyard work and lung cancer could readily result. To minimize this possibility, interviewers were trained to be neutral observers, close-ended rather than open-ended questions were asked, and 10% of interviews were independently verified.

Selection bias could have occurred if knowledge of a person's occupation was used in identifying persons with lung cancer. This was avoided by selecting cases only on the basis of their diagnosis.

Confounding by cigarette smoking was possible if shipyard workers smoked more than did nonshipyard workers. However, by stratifying on smoking as in Table 9.12, smoking was controlled in the analysis.

Based on the results of these two studies, it cannot be said with certainty that asbestos in the absence of cigarette smoke is or is not a lung carcinogen. The data upon which such a judgment would be based are simply too sparse. It would be of considerable value if asbestos by itself were not carcinogenic, for nonsmokers could be hired to work with asbestos. However, since there is no reason to believe that asbestos leads to improved health, exposure to asbestos should be minimized for all persons.

These two studies illustrate some of the practical realities of epidemiologic studies. The study of insulation workers was a prospective cohort study. This was necessary because the study was designed to determine the lung cancer experience in relation to asbestos exposure and smoking. No past information existed on smoking habits or in a cohort of insulation workers; therefore a retrospective cohort study could not be done. The study started in 1967 and, 10 years later, the data on lung cancer among nonsmokers are marginal as to size.

In contrast, the study of lung cancer in relation to prior shipyard work was completed in several years. The number of persons with lung cancer was greater than the number in the cohort study. Cigarette smoking histories were readily obtained. However, the number of persons who had worked in shipyards was only 175. Very little detail was available as to amount of exposure to asbestos. The relatively weak association between lung cancer and shipyard work may only reflect the fact that many shipyard workers were not exposed to asbestos.

D. Beryllium and Respiratory Cancer

In the 1930s and 1940s, respiratory effects of beryllium were first reported.[30] Acute beryllium disease is essentially a pneumonitis that may be severe and lead to death.[31] Chronic beryllium disease is a granulomatous disease resembling sarcoidosis. Symptoms may not develop for several years after exposure to beryllium has ceased. It has been hypothesized that chronic beryllium disease represents an autoimmune response in certain workers.[33]

In 1978 an excess of lung cancer was reported to have occurred among a group of beryllium workers.[33] Earlier versions of this report were challenged by representatives of the beryllium industry and by others.[34,35] These challenges were rebuffed.[36]

The relevant data are presented in Tables 9.13 and 9.14. As seen in Table 9.13, 47 deaths from lung cancer were observed and 34.3 were expected. The excess occurred mainly among men who worked fewer than 5 years; no excess was seen until at least 15 years after onset of exposure. A similar pattern was seen for nonneoplastic respiratory disease (Table 9.14).

Interpretation of these data must take into account not only the comments of the authors and their critics but also general problems associated with all epidemiologic studies. The decision as to whether beryllium is carcinogenic in humans should not be based solely on this one study, but also must take into account other sources of scientific data. Actions to be taken to protect persons who work with beryllium must take into account not only the results of scientific studies, but also must involve negotiation with persons whose primary concern is financial. Since none of these steps is based on an absolute process, the ultimate setting of standards of exposure must be recognized as a political rather than a scientific process.

1. Interpretation of Study Data[33]
a. Comments of Critics[34,35]
1. Cigarette smoking and geographic location of the plant were not adequately

Table 9.13

OBSERVED/EXPECTED DEATHS FROM
LUNG CANCER AMONG BERYLLIUM
WORKERS ACCORDING TO YEARS OF
EXPOSURE AND YEARS SINCE ONSET
OF EXPOSURE[a]

Years of exposure	Years since onset of exposure			
	<15	15—24	25 +	Total
<5	8/8.0	15/11.6	17/9.1[b]	40/28.6[b]
5 +	1/1.5	3/2.5	3/1.7	7/5.7
Total	9/9.4	18/14.1	20/10.8[b]	47/34.3[b]

[a] Expected deaths computed on the basis of age-time specific lung cancer mortality rates for U.S. white males.

[b] Significant at $p < 0.05$.

Table 9.14

OBSERVED/EXPECTED DEATHS
FROM NONNEOPLASTIC
RESPIRATORY DISEASE,
EXCLUDING INFLUENZA AND
PNEUMONIA, AMONG BERYLLIUM
WORKERS ACCORDING TO YEARS
OF EXPOSURE AND YEARS SINCE
ONSET OF EXPOSURE[a]

Years of exposure	Years since onset of exposure			
	<15	15—24	25 +	Total
<5	6/3.6	11/6.4	12/5.6[b]	29/15.6[c]
5 +	1/0.7	1/1.4	0/1.2	2/3.2
Total	7/4.2	12/7.8	12/6.8	31/18.8[b]

[a] Expected deaths computed on the basis of age-time specific mortality rates for U.S. white males.

[b] Significant at $p < 0.05$.

[c] Significant at $p < 0.01$.

taken into account and could account for the apparent excess of lung cancer.

2. If the expected number of lung cancer deaths is corrected for plant location and smoking, the excess is not statistically significant.

3. Mortality rates for 1965—67 were used to estimate the number of deaths expected from lung cancer in 1968—75.[33] Since lung cancer is increasing with time, the expected number of deaths is underestimated.

b. Comments of Authors[33,34,36]

1. Relative to the general population, more beryllium workers were nonsmokers but

more were relatively heavy smokers. It was estimated that at most the lung cancer risk among beryllium workers was increased by 14% by smoking. The overall excess was 37% (Table 9.13).

2. The use of U.S. mortality rates rather than those for the county of residence overestimated the expected number of deaths from lung cancer by 19%.

3. Earlier studies of beryllium workers showed no excess of lung cancer because sufficient time had not passed for exposed persons to develop and die from the disease.

c. Comment

1. The question as to whether the excess of lung cancer among beryllium workers is due to confounding by cigarette smoking or place of residence is difficult to resolve. I do not find this argument to be persuasive, but neither can I demonstrate that the argument is fallacious. The general question as to whether an association is due to confounding bias is one which pervades epidemiologic data. In general, it is unusual for an association to be demonstrated to be due entirely to confounding.

2. For most diseases, mortality rates are changing only slightly with time; therefore use of rates of 1965 to 67 for computing expected numbers in 1968 to 75 should introduce only a trivial error. However, lung cancer rates are rising rapidly with time (about 2%/year). Therefore, correction should be made to the expected numbers for 1968 to 75 to account for the use of earlier rates.

3. Among nonneoplastic respiratory diseases, there were 17 deaths from influenza and pneumonia observed and 21.1 expected.[33] For other diseases in this rubric, there were 31 observed and 18.8 expected (Tables 9.14). The separation of these two types of nonneoplastic respiratory diseases can be defended on the grounds that beryllium disease is generally not coded as pneumonia. However, persons with chronic respiratory disease may die from an acute respiratory process and may be coded as dying from pneumonia. Thus had there also been an excess of death from pneumonia, the authors could have made a legitimate argument for combining the two subcategories of nonmalignant respiratory disease. Clearly, inspection of the data prior to publication and selection of what appears to be relevant is a proper function of the investigator. However, this selection clearly has an influence on sample size and therefore on statistical significance. I find it difficult to attach any interpretive meaning to "$p < 0.01$".

2. Interpretation of Data on Carcinogenicity of Beryllium
a. Consistency

An excess of lung cancer has been reported in three other independent reports.[36] Each of these studies can be criticized for methodologic reasons, as can all epidemiologic studies. In none of the studies is there a large number of men with lung cancer; thus the excesses are quite unstable.

The consistency of findings of an excess occurrence of lung cancer among beryllium workers, while present, is not persuasive.

b. Specificity

In addition to excesses of lung cancer and nonneoplastic respiratory diseases, an excess of fatal cardiovascular disease was also reported among beryllium workers.[33] While pulmonary disease can induce cardiac disease, the effect of beryllium on the human organism is not highly specific.

The lack of specificity of the apparent effects of beryllium does not weaken the belief that it is harmful.

c. Strength of Association

The association between beryllium work and lung cancer overall is weak (SMR = 137). However, the SMR after 25 years or more of the interim is 185 (20/10.8). Confounding could readily account for the overall SMR, but seems unlikely to be the reason for the SMR of 185.

d. Dose-Response Relationship

If years of exposure to a beryllium factory can be taken as a rough measure of dose, there is an inverse relationship between exposure and excess disease (Tables 9.13 and 9.14). However, many of the short-term workers probably had the highest acute exposures to beryllium.[33]

The absence of a clearly measured dose-response relationship between beryllium exposure and lung cancer does not weaken the belief that beryllium may be carcinogenic in man. At worst, the measurement of dose is totally inadequate and no data on dose-response exist.

e. Coherence

Beryllium exposure causes lung cancer in a number of different species of animals.[33] Thus, for this reason alone, there is reason to suspect that it may be carcinogenic in man. Beryllium exposure causes nonneoplastic respiratory disease in man.[30-32] Thus, for this reason alone, there is reason to suspect that it may also cause neoplastic lung disease. While it is unusual for a carcinogen to produce cancer among persons with exposure if only one or more years, it has been suggested that beryllium produces an autoimmune disease.[32] There may be a subgroup of humans who are rendered susceptible to other lung carcinogens by only a brief exposure to beryllium. As in the hypothesized asbestos-smoking relationship, a short period of exposure to beryllium may render the lung of some persons highly susceptible to the carcinogenic potential of cigarette smoke.

A number of coherent (believable) arguments can be constructed to support the hypothesis that beryllium causes lung cancer in man. However, these arguments are based more on thought than on data collected from humans, and thus are peripheral to the epidemiologic issue. Certainly, these coherent arguments do not weaken the hypothesis that beryllium is carcinogenic in man.

f. Temporal Relationship

Among men first employed in the beryllium industry in 1950 or later, there is no excess nonneoplastic respiratory disease or heart disease (Table 9.15).[33] This supports the belief that controls instituted in the 1940s reduced the nonneoplastic effects of beryllium exposure. However, for lung cancer, an excess of lung cancer is also seen in men who started working in 1950 or later (SMR = 152).[33]

The data on temporal relationship do not support the belief that controls instituted in the 1940s have prevented excess cases of lung cancer among persons exposed only since 1950. However, the number of excess cases observed is small and therefore unstable.

g. Statistical Significance

Depending upon the argument used, the occurrence of 47 cases of lung cancer among those beryllium workers may or may not be statistically significantly more than the

Table 9.15
OBSERVED AND EXPECTED
DEATHS FROM SELECTED
DISEASES AMONG BERYLLIUM
WORKERS ACCORDING TO YEAR
OF FIRST EXPOSURE

| | Year of first exposure | | | |
| | <1950 | | ≥1950 | |
Disease	Obs.	Exp.	Obs.	Exp.
Heart	363	313.6	33	35.8
Nonneoplastic respiratory, excluding influenza and pneumonia	31	16.7	0	2.0
Lung cancer	40	29.7	7	4.6

number expected. Whether "$p = 0.04$" or "$p = 0.06$" hardly seems to be of major significance in interpreting these data. Certainly, if in truth the p-value is 0.06, this cannot be taken as support for a nonexcess of lung cancer. At best, it only indicates sparseness of data.

As indicated throughout this discussion, the major concerns with these data are with the way they were collected and analyzed. The presence or absence of statistical significance should have no role in the interpretation of the data.

3. The Setting of a Standard of Exposure to Beryllium

In the 1940s, the standard of exposure to beryllium was set at 2 $\mu g/m^3$; in 1975 NIOSH proposed that the standard be lowered to 0.5 $\mu g/m^3$; industry argued that the lower standard was technically impossible and scientifically unwarranted.[34]

On the basis of the data in Table 9.15, it can be argued that the standard of 2.0 $\mu g/m^3$ has prevented excess deaths from heart disease and nonneoplastic respiratory disease, but has not prevented excess deaths from lung cancer. Clearly, this argument is tenuous. It does not seem rational to spend many millions of dollars on the basis of an excess of 2.4 deaths from lung cancer. Any number of arguments can be raised in objection to the proposed standard.

However, equally tenuous is the belief that the current standard of 2 $\mu g/m^3$ is safe. There is no question that beryllium exposure produces nonneoplastic respiratory disease and little question that it affects the cardiovascular system. Some standard is essential. That standard should be as low as is possible.

The conflict in the setting of a standard of exposure to any industrial substance is straightforward: the cost in human health vs. the cost in dollars. These costs are not independent; a harmful substance produces dollar costs and a safe standard produces dollar savings. However, the data used to balance the health and dollar costs are imperfect; therefore no scientific method can be used to arrive at an optimum standard.

Thus the setting of a beryllium standard is essentially political. Judgments must be made of the data on health and on the persons who produce those data. Those judgments must be made by persons who are not experts in occupational epidemiology and/or beryllium production.

The setting of standards of exposure to industrial and environmental substances is one of the most important problems currently facing society. The adverse effects of occupational exposures and of pollutants are real. It is essential that industry take the lead in controlling both internal exposure to workers and external exposure to the environment. The cost of control must be built into the cost of doing business. The role of the occupational epidemiologist must evolve into that of a person who assists in the setting of standards of exposure rather than that of a person who measures adverse effects of exposure.

E. Summary

Many substances used in industry have been shown to be carcinogenic to exposed workers. The prevention of future excess cases of cancer must rely heavily on nonepidemiologic information. If a substance is known to be a carcinogen in animals, it must be presumed to be a carcinogen in humans. The absence of firm epidemiologic evidence should not weigh heavily as an argument against human carcinogenicity.

Most of the epidemiologic data available as to the carcinogenicity of a substance in humans is based on exposure of 20 to 50 years ago. It is likely that industrial hygiene practices in general are better today than they were yesterday. If some substance has been used for 50 years with no evidence that it is carcinogenic in animals or humans, it seems reasonable to assume that it is not carcinogenic.

In such a situation standards of exposure for today need not be substantially better than those of yesterday. This is not to say that standards be relaxed or that vigilance not be maintained. However, the priority given to controlling such a substance can be relatively low.

Major attention must be given to substances that are newly introduced in industry. Any adverse human effects such as cancer will not be known for several decades. It makes no sense to wait for a demonstrated adverse effect before controlling exposure. Any new substance should be presumed to be harmful and should be controlled. If acute adverse effects appear, no matter how minor they seem, more serious chronic adverse effects must be presumed. Cigarette smoking produces acute bronchitis and lung cancer. Vinyl chloride produces acro-osteolysis and angiosarcoma. Beryllium produces pneumonitis and possibly lung cancer. No newly-introduced substances should be added to this list.

IV. OCCUPATIONAL EXPOSURE TO BENZENE AND LEUKEMIA

Whereas the cause of the majority of cases of lung cancer is known to be cigarette smoking, the cause of the majority of cases of leukemia is unknown. In spite of the predominant role of smoking in the cause of lung cancer, a number of occupational exposures have also been found to produce lung cancer. However, for most cases of leukemia, no occupational cause can be identified.

Leukemia is a cancer of the bone marrow that spreads throughout the blood. For many years, benzene has been known on clinical grounds to poison the bone marrow and lead to aplastic anemia.[37] Common occupations with high exposure to benzene were shoemaking and rotogravure printing. Of 66 persons in these and other industries with acute benzene hemopathy, 11 developed leukemia.[37] While these data derive simply from the clinical setting and have no comparison data, leukemia is a very unusual disease. There is no question that this is an excess of leukemia.

The cases of leukemia among shoemakers and rotogravure workers occurred among persons with very high exposure to benzene. Even though the acute toxic effects of benzene have been known since the early part of this century, workers continued to be exposed to several hundred ppm of benzene.[37] It was among these workers in several

European industries that benzene-attributed leukemia was reported. In the U.S., standards of exposure ranged from 100 ppm in 1941 to 10 ppm in 1971.[38] It was presumed that adherence to these standards would prevent any adverse health effects of benzene.

In 1977 an excess occurrence of leukemia was reported among a group of American workers who were initially exposed to benzene between 1940 and 1949.[38] Out of 140 deaths known to have occurred among 748 pliofilm workers, seven deaths from leukemia were observed in contrast to 1.4 expected on the basis of U.S. white male mortality rates. On the basis of sampling done in 1946 and subsequently, it was judged that the level of benzene did not exceed the exposure standard and probably was 10 to 15 ppm. Largely on the basis of this study, the Emergency Temporary Standard for benzene was set at 1 ppm.[39]

In another study, the mortality experience of 594 workers who were exposed to benzene was reported.[40] The level of exposure to benzene had been measured periodically between 1944 and 1974. The levels of exposure ranged to several hundred ppm, but the averages were estimated to be perhaps 10 to 20 ppm. Two persons died from leukemia in contrast to 1.0 expected. If anything, these persons worked in plant areas with relatively low exposure to leukemia.

In contrast to beryllium, there seems to be little question that benzene has the potential to cause cancer in humans. The data that derive from the clinical setting indicate that high levels of benzene produce both aplastic anemia and leukemia. However, data from the epidemiologic setting are conflicting. In one study of workers exposed to levels of benzene within acceptable standards, an excess of leukemia is seen; in a second study of workers exposed to similar levels, any excess is marginal.

As with beryllium, the setting of the current standard of exposure must be conservative. If a standard of 1 ppm results in no major economic disruption, it clearly is indicated. Even if new costs are involved, it seems prudent to behave as if exposure to 10 ppm of benzene for many years will lead to an excess occurrence of leukemia.

On the other hand, it may be argued that if 10 ppm of benzene is indeed leukemogenic, why has it taken so long to make this determination? Benzene has been used in industry since at least 1900 and thousands of workers have been exposed to levels that likely were several hundred ppm. Since the role of benzene in the etiology of aplastic anemia has been known since at least the 1920s, one might expect that workers exposed to benzene would be monitored for other adverse effects, including leukemia.

Unfortunately, common sense arguments such as this must play a relatively weak role in the setting of standards. While it might be expected that exposure to benzene in the early part of this century was very high, no data exist. While it might be expected that if this exposure led to leukemia it would have been noted before now, no data exist. In the absence of data to the contrary, current standards must err on the side of safety. Future standards must rely on data that are collected today.

V. OCCUPATION AND CARDIOVASCULAR DISEASE

Cancer is comprised of a number of abnormal growths of specific types of tissue in specific locations of the body. Specific types of cancer occur at a low rate. Many cancers are rapidly fatal. For these reasons, the epidemiologic evaluation of the relationship between occupation and cancer can rely heavily on death certificate data and comparisons with rates derived from general populations.

In contrast, cardiovascular disease tends to be systemic, nonspecific and nonfatal. Most of us will develop some type of cardiovascular disease; while many of us will eventually die from cardiovascular disease, the precise mechanism leading to death will be unclear. For these reasons, the epidemiologic evaluation of the relationship between

Table 9.16

DEATH RATES FROM CORONARY HEART DISEASE
(CHD) AMONG SAN FRANCISCO LONGSHOREMEN
ACCORDING TO LEVEL OF WORK ACTIVITY AND
AGE

Work activity level	Age	Person-years of work ($\times 10^3$)	Death rates from CHD per 10,000 person-years	Rate ratio
Heavy	35—44	8.3	4.8	1.0
	45—54	11.0	18.3	1.0
	55—64	7.4	46.2	1.0
	65—74	1.0	76.6	1.0
	All[a]	27.7	26.9	1.0
Moderate	35—44	2.9	6.9	1.4
	45—54	8.7	40.4	2.2
	55—64	9.2	66.1	1.4
	65—74	0.7	136.4	1.8
	All[a]	21.5	46.3	1.7
Light	35—44	3.0	3.3	0.7
	45—54	8.9	30.2	1.7
	55—64	14.5	84.1	1.8
	65—74	17.1	161.2	2.1
	All[a]	43.5	49.0	1.8

[a]   Age-adjusted by the direct method to the 1960 age distribution of California white males.

occupation and cardiovascular disease is subject to much bias and random misclassification. If possible, studies of the association between occupation and cardiovascular disease should rely on internal rather than external comparisons. Such comparisons can be based on data that are collected primarily by the investigator and thus are comparable among groups. Further, measures of morbidity as well as measures of mortality may be utilized.

A. Mortality from Coronary Heart Disease among Longshoremen

In 1951, longshoremen in San Francisco were enrolled into a prospective cohort study.[41] As part of the study, the energy output required by each person's job was measured annually. Three levels of energy expenditure were defined: heavy, moderate, and light. Persons who died from coronary artery disease between 1951 and 1972 were categorized as to their level of energy expenditure on the June prior to their death. Persons who died after retirement were categorized as being at the light level of energy expenditure. As seen in Table 9.16, the death rate from coronary heart disease among men whose work was the heaviest was 60% of that among men whose work activity was moderate or light.

This association could be disputed on the ground that men in good cardiovascular health tend to enter the heavy level of work activity; however, all longshoremen were considered to be healthy on employment. It might be argued that as cardiovascular disease develops, men selectively transfer to a less strenuous level of activity; however, this potential problem was minimized by using the work activity level approximately 6 months before death. Further, the association was stronger if only sudden death was considered. It might be argued that men with heavy work activity smoked fewer cigarettes or otherwise had been potential for good cardiovascular health; the lower death rate among those with heavy work activity persisted when control was performed for cigarette smoking, blood pressure, weight, previous heart disease, and glucose metabolism.

For two primary reasons, the analysis of these data was conducted using internal directly standardized comparisons rather than external indirectly standardized comparisons.

1.   Causes of deaths compared among levels of work activity were coronary artery disease and sudden death. Each of these diseases is subject to a high degree of subjectivity in definition. In an internal comparison, this uncertainty as to diagnosis could lead only to random misclassification. Any differences between work activity level group could not be attributed to this uncertainty. However, if an external comparison had been made with published mortality rate for CHD, substantial coding or certification differences may have been present.

2.   In these data, age is strongly associated with work activity and with coronary disease mortality (Table 9.16). "Heavy" workers tend to be young and "light" workers tend to be old. Further, there is a definite trend with age in the rate ratio comparing light to heavy workers. An SMR type of indirect standardization would not control completely for this age difference.

B. Carbon Disulfide and Coronary Heart Disease

In 1967, two cohorts of workers in Finland were enrolled into a prospective cohort study.[42] The exposed cohort was 343 men who had been exposed to carbon disulfide in a viscose rayon plant for at least 5 years. The control cohort was 343 paper workers from the same town who were matched to the exposed on age, birth district, and similarity of work. Mortality from 6/1/67 through 12/31/72 was observed.

Death from coronary heart disease is presented in Table 9.17. In the internal comparison of the 5½ year attack rates, coronary-artery disease occurred over five times as frequently among the viscose rayon workers as among the paper workers. It is unknown whether the rate among viscose rayon workers is too high or whether the rate among paper workers is too low. However, in the external comparison with Finnish death rates, it can be seen that each is the case. The rate of coronary heart disease among viscose rayon workers is higher than that among the general population, and the rate among paper workers is lower.

In this example, the ratio of the two SMRs (5.3) is essentially the same as the rate ratio obtained in a direct comparison of the viscose rayon workers and the paper workers. This is a direct result of the study design: the age distribution of the two groups of workers was made to be equal. Therefore, in the computation of the SMRs, the same weights were used for each group in weighing the age-specific rates of the Finnish male general population.

In addition to data on mortality from coronary heart disease, data also were collected on morbidity.[43] The viscose rayon workers also had excesses of nonfatal myocardial infarctions, of angina pectoris, of "coronary" electrocardiograms, and of high systolic blood pressure.

C. Comment

In each of these studies an association is seen between cardiovascular disease mortality and occupation. In the longshoremen study the association is negative; in the viscose rayon worker study the association is positive. In the longshoreman study only

Table 9.17
DEATHS FROM CORONARY HEART DISEASE (CHD) AMONG FINNISH VISCOSE RAYON WORKERS AND AMONG CONTROLS

Internal Comparison

	Coronary heart disease death			
Exposure	Yes	No	Total	Rate
Yes	16	327	343	4.7/100
No	3	340	343	0.9/100

Rate ratio = 4.7/0.9 = 5.2

External Comparison

	Coronary heart disease death		
Exposure	Observed	Expected[a]	Obs/Exp (SMR)
Yes	16	7.8	2.1
No	3	8.1	0.4

Ratio of two SMRs = 2.1/0.4 = 5.3

[a] Expected deaths based on age-specific mortality rates for Finnish males.

directly standardized internal comparisons were made; in the viscose rayon study both internal and external comparisons were made.

There are only a few studies in which a clear-cut association has been found between work and cardiovascular disease. This probably is a reflection both of biology and of methodology. Most cardiovascular disease probably occurs for reasons unrelated to a person's occupation. The rate ratio of work-related cardiovascular disease is therefore low. Also, the imprecision of definition of cardiovascular disease tends to minimize any measure of association with work.

Routine epidemiologic surveillance of industrial groups has the potential to be a valuable source of data on cardiovascular disease. On entrance into a work population and periodically thereafter, information can be obtained on factors of importance in the development of cardiovascular disease. Relatively precise measures can be obtained of occupational exposures; relatively accurate measures of cardiovascular disease should be possible through company-related health evaluation and insurance programs. This aspect of an occupational surveillance system can be useful in general preventive medicine as well as in the prevention of occupational diseases.

REFERENCES

1. National Institute for Occupational Safety and Health, Criteria Documents, U.S. Department of Health, Education and Welfare, Washington, D.C., 1972-1979.

2. International Agency for Research on Cancer, *IARC Monographs on the Evaluation of Carcinogenic Risk of Chemicals in Man,* International Agency for Research on Cancer, Lyon, 1974.
3. Infante, P. F., Wagoner, J. K., McMichael, A. J., Waxweiler, R. J., and Falk, H., Genetic risks of vinyl chloride, *Lancet,* 1, 734, 1976.
4. Meyer, M. B., Jonas, B. S., and Tonasci, J. A., Perinatal events associated with maternal smoking during pregnancy, *Am. J. Epidemiol.,* 103, 464, 1976.
5. Infante, P. F., Wagoner, J. K., McMichael, A. J., Waxweiler, R. J., and Falk, H., Genetic risks of vinyl chloride, *Lancet,* 1, 1289, 1976.
6. Fabia, J. and Thuy, T. D., Occupation of father at time of birth of children dying of malignant diseases, *Br. J. Prev. Soc. Med.,* 28, 98, 1974.
7. Hakulinen, T., Salonen, T., and Teppo, L., Cancer in the offspring of fathers in the hydrocarbon-related occupations, *Br. J. Prev. Soc. Med.* 30, 138, 1976.
8. MacMahon, B., Prenatal X-ray and childhood cancer, *J. Nat. Cancer Inst.,* 28, 1173, 1962.
9. Epstein, S., Environmental determinants of human cancer, *Cancer Res.,* 34, 2425, 1974.
10. Doll, R., Cancer of the lung and nose in nickel workers, *Br. J. Ind. Med.,* 15, 217, 1958.
11. Doll, R., Morgan, L. G., and Speizer, F. E., Cancers of the lung and nasal sinuses in nickel workers, *Br. J. Cancer,* 24, 623, 1970.
12. Doll, R., Mathews, J. D., and Morgan, L. G., Cancers of the lung and nasal sinuses in nickel workers: a reassessment of the period of risk, *Br. J. Ind. Med.,* 34, 102, 1977.
13. Sunderman, F. W., The current status of nickel carcinogenesis, *Ann. Clin. Lab. Sci.,* 3, 156, 1973.
14. Pedersen, E., Høgetveit, A. C., and Andersen, A., Cancer of the respiratory organs among workers at a nickel refinery in Norway, *Int. J. Cancer,* 12, 32, 1973.
15. Creech, J. L., Jr. and Johnson, M. N., Angiosarcoma of liver in the manufacture of polyvinyl chloride, *J. Occup. Med.,* 16, 151, 1974.
16. Wegman, D. H., Peters, J. M., Jaeger, R. J., Burgess, W. A., and Boden, L. I., Vinyl chloride: can the worker be protected? *N. Engl. J. Med.,* 294, 653, 1976.
17. Monson, R. R., Peters, J. M. and Johnson, M. N., Proportional mortality among vinyl-chloride workers, *Lancet,* 2, 397, 1974.
18. Duck, B. W., Carter, J. T., and Coombes, E. J., Mortality study of workers in a polyvinyl-chloride production plant, *Lancet,* 2, 1197, 1975.
19. Monson, R. R., Effects of industrial environment on health, *Environ. Law,* 8, 663, 1978.
20. Lloyd, J. W., and Ciocco, A., Long-term mortality study of steelworkers. I. Methodology, *J. Occup. Med.,* 11, 299, 1969.
21. Lloyd, J. W., Lundin, F. E., Jr., Redmond, C. K., and Geiser, P. B., Long-term mortality study of steelworkers. IV. Mortality by work area, *J. Occup. Med.,* 12, 151, 1970.
22. Redmond, C. K., Strobino, B. R., and Cypess, R. H., Cancer experience among coke by-product workers, *Ann. N. Y. Acad. Sci.,* 271, 102, 1976.
23. U.S. Department of Health, Education and Welfare, Criteria for a Recommended Standard on Occupational Exposure to Coke Oven Emissions, DHEW Publ. No. 73-110116, Washington, D.C., 1973.
24. Levine, R. J.,Asbestos — An Information Resource, DHEW Publ. No. (NIH) 78-1681, National Cancer Institute, Department of Health, Education and Welfare, Washington, D.C., 1978.
25. Saracci, R., Asbestos and lung cancer: an analysis of the epidemiological evidence on the asbestos-smoking interaction, *Int. J. Cancer,* 20, 323, 1977.
26. Selikoff, I. J. and Hammond, E. C., Multiple risk factors in environmental cancer, in *Persons at High Risk of Cancer,* Fraumeni, J. F., Jr., Ed., Academic Press, New York, 1975, 467.
27. Selikoff, I. J., Cancer risk of asbestos exposure, in *Origins of Human Cancer,* Hiatt, H. H., Watson, J. D., and Winsten, J. A., Eds., Cold Spring Harbor Laboratory, New York, 1977, 1765.
28. Blot, W. J., Harrington, J. M., Toledo, A., Hoover, R., Heath, C. W., Jr., and Fraumeni, J. F., Jr., Lung cancer after employment in shipyards during World War II, *N. Engl. J. Med.,* 299, 620, 1978.
29. Blot, W. J. and Fraumeni, J. F., Jr., Geographical patterns of lung cancer: industrial correlations, *Am. J. Epidemiol.,* 103, 539, 1976.
30. Hardy, J., Beryllium poisoning — lessons in control of man-made disease, *N. Engl. J. Med.,* 273, 1188, 1965.
31. Hunter, P.,*The Diseases of Occupations,* The English Universities Press, London, 1975, 399.
32. Sterner, J. H. and Eisenbud, M., Epidemiology of beryllium intoxication, *Arch. Ind. Hyg. Occup. Med.,* 4, 123, 1951.
33. Wagoner, J. K., Infante, P. F., and Bayliss, D. L., Beryllium: an etiologic agent in the induction of lung cancer, non-neoplastic respiratory disease, and heart disease among industrially exposed workers, *Environ. Res.,* 21, 15, 1980.

34. **Shapley, D.,** Occupational cancer: government challenged in beryllium proceedings, *Science,* 198, 898, 1977.
35. **Eisenbud, M., Goldwater, L. J., Higgins, I., MacMahon, B., Rogers, A. E., Roth, H. D., Tabershaw, I. R., van Ordstrand, H. S., Cooper, W. C., and McLean, A. A.,** AOMA board expresses concern over quality of NIOSH research, *J. Occup. Med.,* 20, 434, 1978.
36. **Wagoner, J. K., Infante, P. F., and Mancuso, T.,** Beryllium: carcinogenicity studies, *Science,* 201, 198, 1978.
37. **Vigliani, E. C.,** Leukemia associated with benzene exposure, *Ann. N. Y. Acad. Sci.,* 271, 143, 1976.
38. **Infante, P. F., Rinsky, R. A., Wagoner, J. K., and Young, R. J.,** Leukemia in benzene workers, *Lancet,* 2, 76, 1977.
39. **Occupational Safety and Health Administration,** Emergency temporary standard for occupational exposure to benzene, *Fed. Regis.,* 42, 22516, 1977.
40. **Ott, M. G., Townsend, J. C., Fishbeck, W. A., and Langner, R. A.,** Mortality among individuals occupationally exposed to benzene, *Arch. Environ. Health,* 33, 3, 1978.
41. **Paffenbarger, R. S. Jr. and Hale, W. E.,** Work activity and coronary heart mortality, *N. Engl. J. Med.,* 292, 545, 1975.
42. **Hernberg, S., Nurminen, M., and Tolonen, M.,** Excess mortality from coronary heart disease in viscose rayon workers exposed to carbon disulfide, *Work Environ. Health,* 10, 93, 1973.
43. **Tolonen, M., Hernberg, S., Nurminen, M., and Tiitola, K.,** A follow-up study of coronary heart disease in viscose rayon workers exposed to carbon disulphide, *Br. J. Ind. Med.,* 32, 1, 1975.

Epilogue

INDUSTRY AND THE ENVIRONMENT

Potential adverse effects of exposure to substances used in industry are not limited to persons who are occupationally exposed. Chemicals used within the plant are released in the form of solid, liquid, and gaseous discharges. Some of these discharges contribute to the pollution of land, water, and air. There is concern that the resultant pollution may cause adverse effects on human health.

The methods used in occupational epidemiology can be adapted to the study of the relationship between the environment and health. However, the task will be considerably more difficult. Few populations exist that can be defined on the basis of environmental exposure. The level of exposure to chemicals in the environment is many times lower than the level within industry. The collection of data on health from general populations cannot rely on any ongoing surveillance systems.

For these reasons, the assessment of health and disease within working populations is especially important to the health of the general population. Harmful exposures that are identified within occupational groups can be controlled within and outside of the industrial environment. The future of the occupational epidemiologist will lie in the protection of the health of the workers, their families, and their neighbors.

TERMINOLOGY

The words used to describe the various components in the collection and analysis of epidemiologic data are based on daily expressions. Because of this, a number of different terms are used by different epidemiologists to describe the same thing. This leads to disagreement. More serious is the fact that the same word may be used to describe different things. This leads to confusion.

In this book I have tried to be internally consistent and to use terms that bear some logical relationship to each other. In so doing, I have coined some phrases that I do not use on a daily basis. In some instances I have given alternate words or expressions that are in common use. While there are current efforts to codify epidemiologic terminology, no generally accepted words and definitions are at hand.

ASSOCIATION	— Two variables are associated if one is more (or less) common in the presence of the second.
ATTRIBUTABLE RISK	— See Rate Difference.
BIAS	— An error in the measure of the association between two variables.
CASE-CONTROL STUDY	— Selection of study groups to be compared based on presence or absence of disease.
CAUSE	— An exposure is a cause if, by modification of the exposure, the rate of disease is altered.
COHORT STUDY	— Selection of study groups to be compared based on presence or absence of exposure.
CONFOUNDING BIAS	— A (potential) attribute of data. In measuring an association between an exposure and a disease, a confounding factor is one that is associated with the exposure and independently is a cause of the disease. Confounding bias can be controlled if information on the confounding factor is present.
CROSS-SECTIONAL	— The time sequence between exposure and disease cannot be inferred.
DISEASE	— A (potential) result of exposure.
EXPERIMENTAL STUDY	— A study in which the entrance of an individual into the exposed or nonexposed study group is determined by the investigator.
EXPOSURE	— A (potential) cause of disease.
INCIDENCE RATE	— Number of new cases of disease per unit of population per unit of time, e.g., 3/1000/year.
INFORMATION BIAS	— See Observation Bias.
LONGITUDINAL	— The time sequence between exposure and disease can be inferred.
MATCHING	— A procedure to reduce the biasing effect of a confounding variable. A feature of selection to study groups.
OBSERVATION BIAS (INFORMATION BIAS)	— An attribute of data collection. In the collection of data from two groups (cases, controls; exposed, nonexposed) observation bias occurs when noncomparable methods of data collection are used.

ODDS RATIO	— An estimation or equivalent of rate ratio. The odds of having the disease among the exposed divided by the odds of having the disease among the nonexposed.
PREVALENCE RATE	— Number of existent cases of disease per unit of population, e.g., 5/100.
PROSPECTIVE	— A study characteristic. Disease has *not* occurred in study groups at start of study.
RANDOM MISCLASSIFICA-TION	— Imprecise categorization of a person as exposed or nonexposed or as diseased or nondiseased. Random misclassification can only alter the rate ratio toward 1.0.
RANDOMIZATION	— A procedure to reduce the confounding effects of many confounding variables simultaneously. A feature of assignment to exposure or nonexposure group.
RATE	— Quantity or degree of a thing measured per unit of something else (Webster's New Collegiate Dictionary). In epidemiology, number of cases per unit of population.
RATE DIFFERENCE	— One rate minus another rate with the same dimensions. The units correspond to those of the rates.
RATE RATIO	— One rate divided by another rate with the same dimensions. A unitless measure of association.
RELATIVE RISK	— See Rate Ratio.
RETROSPECTIVE	— A study characteristic. Disease has already occurred in study groups at start of study.
SELECTION BIAS	— An attribute of study group definition. In a case-control study, selection bias may result if knowledge of exposure is used in defining study groups. In a cohort study, selection bias may result if knowledge of disease is used in defining study groups.
STANDARDIZATION	— A procedure to reduce the biasing effect of a confounding variable. A feature of data analysis.
STANDARDIZED MORTALITY RATIO	— The ratio of mortality rates, expressed as a percentage, usually adjusted for age and/or time differences between the two groups being compared.
STANDARDIZED PROPORTIONAL MORTALITY RATIO	— The ratio of two mortality proportions, expressed as a percentage, usually adjusted for age and/or time differences between the two groups being compared.
STATISTICAL SIGNIFICANCE	— A measure of the stability of the measure of an association.
STRATIFICATION	— A procedure to reduce the biasing effect of a confounding variable. A feature of data analysis.

Index

INDEX